The following is a series of text messages

DAY 1 – Thursday, September 7, 2017

> *1:47 pm, conversation between my sister and me.*

ᒣ Kelly: Scott and I just got contacted by the hospital about Rachel. They were looking to contact you. Did they get you? Is everything OK?

> ᒣ Me: Yes. I'm headed there now. She's in ICU that's all I know. I will keep you posted. Will you call dad for me?

ᒣ Kelly: Ok. I'll let him know. Love you both! If you need anything, please let us know.

> *1:48 pm, message to 2 friends.*
> ᒣ Me: Rachel's in ICU at the hospital. They just called me and told me to come.

ᒣ Beth: Oh dear lord!!! Thank goodness they got a hold of you. Did they tell you any details? Keep me posted. 🙏 Love you.

ᒣ Nancy: An overdose? Car wreck? Prayers

> *2:30 pm, conversation between me and my daughter, Rachel's sister.*
> ᒣ Me: Rachel's in ICU. I think it's similar to your friend Britlie's situation when she got so sick.

ᒣ Maddy: Wait what?? When are u gonna go see her?

⅃ Me: I'm here now. She's not conscious. She has a ton of tubes and stuff. They're running a bunch of tests. She has massive infection throughout her body. She has sepsis. Her organs are affected. She has a growth on at least 1 heart valve that will probably mean surgery. I'm waiting on test results to see exactly what treatment will be.

⅃ Maddy: Omg keep me posted! I'll be home tonight.

⅃ Me: Good. I could use help with Z.

⅃ Maddy: Will I be able to come to the hospital?

⅃ Me: Yes. During visiting hours there can be 3 people. I have a pass that will allow one of us to be here anytime. Right now she's not aware of anything. She didn't have any ID on her. They were able to get her to say her name and they found her on social media and found me that way. They also called Aunt Kelly and Uncle Scott looking for relatives. They already knew about Daddy's death from one of her Facebook posts.

⅃ Maddy: Where did they pick her up at?

⅃ Me: Somewhere on the west side I think. They found her on the street.

⅃ Maddy: Oh okk. How long are u gonna be there?

⅃ Me: Not sure. They can't get the catheter in and she just peed the bed.

⅃ Maddy: Okk. When I come in town I'm gonna call u and see where ur and then I wanna see Rachel tonight if u can give me the pass.

⌐ Me: It's really cold in here so dress warm.

3:24 pm
⌐ Me: Wow! They have a ton of questions. I've talked to the nurse and the social worker and admissions. I had to try to remember Rachel's complete medical history. I'm afraid I have forgotten to tell them something.

⌐ Kelly: If you think of something later just tell them. What did they ask?

⌐ Me: About any previous surgeries, illnesses or allergies. How long she's been using. If she's married or has any children. Some things about her private life I feel bad I don't even know. I mean I know she's not married and I know she has no children, but I don't know if she has a boyfriend. I said I think she started using heroine about 5 years ago, at around 23.

⌐ Kelly: How is she? Did you get to talk to her?

⌐ Me: I'm in with her, but she's not really conscious enough to talk.

⌐ Kelly: Thankfully she's there now getting treatment. That's so scary, but she's a strong girl. It will just take some time.

⌐ Me: I know. Aside from what I told you, we are still waiting on test results.

↲ Me: They gave me a clear drawstring bag with all of her possessions in it- nasty, dirty clothes and a black mini backpack. This bothers me. I want them to know that she's not just some homeless person. I explained to them that I had given her a choice. If she wanted to stay at home she had to be in treatment so she left. I told them about her rehab history. She's got a family that loves her and we have been trying to help her.

↲ Kelly: She is loved. We know that. Keep me posted.

↲ Me: I will.

6:48 pm, continued simultaneous conversations between me and 2 friends.

↲ Me: Here's what I know so far. She was found on the street somewhere on the west side. The police brought her to the ER as a Jane Doe. She was semi-conscious and somehow they got her to say her name and they looked her up on Facebook to find her people. They actually called my sister and brother in law first. She arrived at the ER around 5 a.m. and was moved to ICU a couple hours later.

↲ Beth: How is she now???? Is she still in there?

↲ Me: She has a massive infection throughout her body that affects all of her organs, sepsis. They did a CAT scan and say she has had several small strokes. She has a growth on at least one of her heart valves that will require surgery. They will do a heart probe in the morning if her platelet levels are up. Her blood pressure is extremely low and they have had to give her something to bring it up. She is still semi-conscious and incoherent. She kind of wakes up and cries but then goes right back out. She's not making any sense. She is still in ICU. I finally came home to take care of the animals but they will call if anything changes.

↲ Beth: Oh wow! That's really too bad BUT you know, this could be the blessing we've been waiting for. Maybe once this settles down, she'll be largely detoxed and she'll be so scared she'll be thankful to be alive and ready to turn her life around. That's what I've been praying for. I've been asking God to scare her so bad that this will be the turning point for her and He can then heal her. Call or text me ANYTIME, I'm here for you.

↲ Me: Thanks! I actually said the exact same thing to one of the nurses. But right now she is extremely sick and we have to pray that she is allowed the chance to turn her life around. She has an uphill battle. The nurse said there is a good chance that this hospital will consider her heart surgery too risky and will send her to another hospital.

↲ Beth: That makes me feel better. I felt kind of guilty asking for someone to be really sick. But we both know that had to happen for anything to change. I hope she can have the surgery here. Memorial is supposed to be one of the best heart hospitals in the country, I heard.

↲ Nancy: I'm so sorry...prayers will continue...

↲ Nancy: Oh, maybe this will be her rock bottom...where's Maddy? She's only got one way to go from here, God be with her and your precious family. I am so so sorry, Maureen 🙏

> ↲ Me: Yes. I know she had to hit rock bottom. I can't imagine anything worse. If this doesn't get her to try, I'll be convinced she's suicidal. Hopefully I'll know more about the heart surgery if they can do the probe in the morning. Maddy was at the beach, but she's on her way home.

↲ Nancy: I truly believe Jesus Christ is her only hope... and that's what I'll pray for.

> ↲ Me: I agree with you. I prayed with her in ICU. I just know some part of her heard me.

↲ Nancy: She did hear. Is she at General? You should stay home tonight...I know that you won't sleep, but you can relax better...you're gonna need your rest with what you have to deal with. When she's more responsive that's when you need to be there. Was your sister with you?

⌐ Me: No but I relayed messages to her and she kept everyone updated. I kind of decided the same thing about staying home tonight. There's nothing I can do right now. She didn't even know I was there. I'll go first thing in the morning and be there as long as I can. It will be easier with Maddy here to help with the animals and take turns with Rachel.

⌐ Nancy: Yes, that's a good plan. Please, keep me posted. Still praying. I'll let my church know to pray. Will ask all prayer warriors.

⌐ Me: Thank you. That would be great!!

8:37 pm
⌐ Me: Ok so one thing I didn't tell you that is really bothering me. Evidently she had injuries that made it difficult to get the catheter in place.

⌐ Beth: Whoa!!! God love her! Did they suspect assault?

⌐ Me: They didn't really say but they had to wait all day to get a specialist there to place it. She peed in the bed 4 times.

⌐ Beth: It's hard to imagine what that poor child has been through.

⌐ Me: I know. She has told me some disturbing things about her time in New Jersey that are too difficult to think about right now, but she had an option. She chose that life over treatment. That's the scariest part. They also said that you get one chance with the surgery. If she relapses and would need surgery again no one will do it. Her heart will just stop beating.

⌐ Beth: Oh crap! Well, this just HAS to scare her straight. It just has to! Surely when she realizes she was on the brink of death and has a second chance, she'll make the right choice. One good thing is she's not aware of what's going on. Hopefully, when she's fully conscious, the drugs will be out of her system, or at least mostly, so the detox won't be so bad and she'll be able to think more clearly. I know she chose this life, but now that the drugs have a hold on her, it's not her doing these things and thinking that way – it's the drugs. Hopefully she'll get a clear head soon. I know she has a looong road ahead, but I'm still hoping and praying she'll make it. I wonder what would happen when she becomes fully cognizant and she would throw a fit and demand to be released from the hospital and refuse all the medical treatment she needs. Could they keep her?

> ⌐ Me: Nope. They couldn't. I signed a paper to act on her behalf until she's able to. Then they have to let her make her own decisions. She's an adult. But I did think of that too. At least she will detox whether she knows it or not. There is a much better chance of reasoning with her once she's clean. Plus, there is a social worker here that said she will do all she can do to get Rachel to accept treatment.

⌐ Beth: That's what I was thinking. Detox while she's out of it, doesn't know it and then when she's clean, she will be easier to talk to and definitely more likely to listen to reason. Thank goodness there's a social worker. That's a plus. What do Maddy and Alex think about all this? Are they doing ok?

꒜ Me: Maddy was at the beach. She's on her way home now. Alex wanted the details but hasn't responded since. He tries to act cool but I think he's probably upset.

꒜ Beth: Oh yes! That's like Samantha. Act like nothing bothers them but roiling on the inside.

꒜ Me: Maddy's the open book. If she has a feeling, she can't hide it!

꒜ Beth: Not to save her soul!

꒜ Me: I still can't believe Rachel was found on the street. Who would just throw her out being that sick?

꒜ Beth: Yes. Discarded like the trash.

꒜ Me: I wonder if they were afraid of the police coming to wherever she was and finding things or if they wanted more drugs for themselves.

꒜ Beth: Maybe both.

꒜ Me: Disgusting! It also breaks my heart for Rachel. She has always been so trusting. I guarantee she thinks those people are her friends.

꒜ Beth: I know. She sees only the good in people and doesn't believe there could be bad.

꒜ Me: She is the perfect target for manipulative people. She takes everything at face value. She has never been able to read between the lines. She bonds with someone that she just assumes is being honest with her and they become almost like family in her mind.

↲ <u>Beth</u>: It's sweet but scary.

↲ <u>Me</u>: It definitely made her vulnerable.

DAY 2 – Friday, September 8, 2017

<u>*10:02 am, conversation between me and a friend.*</u>

⌐ <u>Me</u>: So far not much different. Her breathing is more rapid so they're watching that. She's a little more awake at times and talking a lot more. She recognized me today. Waiting for the Doctor to do the heart tests.

⌐ <u>Beth</u>: That's great she recognized you. And also that she's not fully awake. The longer she's out of it, the more time for and easier the detox and hopefully the more compliant she'll be when it comes time for her to make the right decisions. Let me know as soon as you know anything about the heart tests.

⌐ <u>Me</u>: I will. They ask her questions to check her mental state. They asked her where she was and she said "here". I thought that was a great answer!

⌐ <u>Beth</u>: 😄 😄 That's great! Technically can't argue with that.

⌐ <u>Me</u>: That's what I thought too!

⌐ <u>Me</u>: You know Rachel's one-track mind. She is very thirsty and thoroughly disgusted that they will not give her any water or ice chips. They are afraid she will choke. Every time she opens her eyes she asks for water. One time she rolled over and made an ice crunching face at me!

⌐ <u>Beth</u>: LOL. That's good that she's so determined.

⌐ Me: She asked if she had to beg for water. She actually said in her best beggar's accent, "Please sir, can you spare some water?" I laughed so hard!

⌐ Beth: 😂😂😂

⌐ Me: The nurse said that the longer she is somewhat stable and keeps getting the antibiotics the better her chances are. And the longer time from whatever happened to her, the better.

10:30 am, conversation with a friend.

⌐ Nancy: How's Rachel today?

⌐ Me: She seems a little better. She's talking more.

⌐ Nancy: Prayers continue🙏🙏.

⌐ Me: If you haven't already heard, she's telling everybody that she's thirsty and wants water!

⌐ Nancy: Give the girl some water. What about ice chips?

⌐ Me: They're afraid she'll choke. I wish they would let her try. It's making me thirsty!

11:21 am
⌐ Me: They haven't done the heart test yet but she will need surgery on a large abscess on her arm once they get the infection under control.

⌐ Beth: Yuk. But that sounds like one of the least of her problems. I wonder what actually did happen for them to find her that way. I guess we'll never know.

⅃ Me: The nurse has been asking her if she knows what happened but she can't say much right now. She did tell him multiple times she wanted heroine. She's been here long enough that all of the drug tests come back negative. He is giving her meds so she won't start withdrawing.

⅃ Beth: Great. Have they been able to fight the infection?

⅃ Me: She has multiple IV's. One of them is antibiotic. He said as of right now things are trending the right way.

⅃ Beth: Fantastic! That's a BIGGIE! But DAMN! She's saying she wants heroine? But it's still too soon. Hopefully, she won't after a few days.

⅃ Me: Very true. I agree.

⅃ Me: She has the practiced statement down. She tried to say that she is refusing medical treatment and wants to leave. I told her that if she can unhook herself and walk to go for it.

⅃ Beth: Why on earth would she want to leave?

⅃ Me: I don't think she knows what she's saying. It sounds rehearsed. Like she's been taught to say it.

2:47 pm
⅃ Me: They are putting off the heart tests for a couple of days because the infection is so out of control. Her platelet levels won't come up so they are consulting with a hematologist.

⅃ Beth: Well poop. I thought that was getting better.

⌐ Me: The hematologist is here now.

⌐ Beth: Great! That was fast.

⌐ Me: I didn't really find out anything new. The doctor just kept saying she's very sick and she has a lot going on. She's getting more incoherent again.

⌐ Beth: I wonder why? Is it because of anything they are giving her in the hospital? Did the hematologist say?

⌐ Me: They are not sure if it's because of drugs, the infection or the strokes. The infection is really bad. I don't know what it all means but they have said sepsis, MRSA and serratia. And it's throughout her whole body.

⌐ Beth: MRSA is a bear to treat I've heard. And sepsis is definitely not good.

⌐ Me: They just gave her something for withdrawal symptoms. Hopefully she will settle down a little. She was getting very restless and anxious. New target date for heart test is Monday.

⌐ Beth: Well that will give her a few days to recover a little more. Seems like what she needs now is rest, sleep and more rest.

⌐ Me: I agree. It's hard to tell how long it's been since she had a good rest.

5:00 pm
⌐ Me: Heart test is being put off until Monday. Platelet levels still too low.

↲ Nancy: Is she still doing better? Still talking?

↲ Me: She's pretty much out again. The nurse thinks she may be withdrawing so they gave her something for it.

↲ Nancy: Good…withdrawal must be horrible…and add everything else.

↲ Me: Honestly she's so out of it, it's hard to tell. We could tell she may be having symptoms by how restless she got and started sweating.

↲ Nancy: How are your sisters and parents doing?

↲ Me: They're doing OK, worried of course. I've been talking to them and keeping them updated. They are planning on visiting this evening.

↲ Nancy: That's good….will be good for Rachel too.

↲ Me: Definitely!

7:53 pm, conversation with another sister.
↲ Me: I'm sure Kelly updated you. I'm just sitting here with Rachel.

↲ Colleen: Yes. Anything new?

↲ Me: No. They just did a shift change and I met her nighttime nurse. She seems really nice. Everybody here has been.

↲ Colleen: That's good. She's getting good care.

↲ Me: I think I'm in shock or something. Everything is kind of being thrown at me so fast.

↲ Colleen: I know what you mean.

↲ Me: I'm trying to take in all of the medical stuff. I nod my head when the doctors talk to me, but I have to look up what I can remember after they leave!

↲ Colleen: Lol! I know. It gets confusing.

↲ Me: Then I think, this is Rachel they are talking about. It's hard to put together. She's just another patient to them. Idk. I can't explain it.

↲ Colleen: I get it. It's hard to believe this is happening to her.

↲ Me: Yes. All of it, from the fact that she has addiction issues. I don't know how we got here. She is so smart and creative, so much potential.

↲ Colleen: I know. She has been special from the time she was little. She just has a spark.

↲ Me: I have always thought so too. I was just thinking about the time Brad and I went to Kings Island and you, Dad and Anna were watching Rachel.

↲ Colleen: That was a long time ago. She was just a toddler.

↲ Me: And so spoiled! Remember when you were taking the trash out?

↲ Colleen: Omg! Yes! She said present Rae Rae?

↲ Me: Lol. She just assumed everything was for her!

↲ Colleen: Everything kind of was back then! She was adorable! When do you think all of this started? I mean the drug use.

⅃ Me: I have thought about that a lot during the last 5 years. I've kind of pieced things together through bits of information I have gotten. It was soon after she met RS. She was back from Morgantown and had just started working in catering at the hotel.

⅃ Colleen: I never met him and based on what you've told me I'm glad.

⅃ Me: At first I just thought he was a little rough around the edges but seemed nice enough. He made her happy so I was OK with him. She spent a lot of time with him. Between work and him I really didn't see her that much. Then he got the puppy. That was it. She fell hard.

⅃ Colleen: Awe! I can just imagine. She has such a soft spot for animals.

⅃ Me: Yes, animals and babies. It's her maternal instinct. She has always wanted her own little family unit. I think she saw RS and the puppy that way. Shortly after that they moved in together. Remember that tiny, filthy, disgusting little hole in the wall place?

⅃ Colleen: I remember you telling me about it.

⅃ Me: It's the one that lead to the mental hygiene attempt a few months ago. It was gross. 2 sloppy adults plus a giant dog in a place the size of a closet! It was close enough for her to walk to work. RS did not work. She was working a lot of hours and walking to and from work. You know she has had anxiety issues for a long time. I'm guessing she was pretty stressed out. He started giving her things to calm her down and help her relax.

ॱ Colleen: Oh crap. She knew better.

ॱ Me: I know, that's why as much as I dislike him and wish she never would have met him, I don't blame him. It was her choice. She was still able to keep it together at that point and she always sounded fine when I talked to her on the phone.

ॱ Colleen: OMG! Her little voice. She has always had the sweetest sounding little girl voice.

ॱ Me: Lol! Especially on the phone. Anyway as time went by, the drugs got stronger and more frequent. Maddy told me that Rachel and RS would get in to huge, explosive fights. Eventually he moved out. She called me and was so upset. I went to see her. That's when I knew something was really wrong. She had lost so much weight and just didn't look good.

ॱ Colleen: This part I remember. Cassie had seen her at the mall and told me how thin she was.

ॱ Me: Yes. You warned me, but I think I was in denial. I really thought she was just heart-broken, which she was. She's very loyal. Once she's attached to someone, she just can't say goodbye. I think that's part of her personality but made stronger by losing her dad. I wanted her to move back home, but she refused. I think she was hoping he and the dog would come back.

ॱ Colleen: He did though, didn't he?

⌐ Me: He did briefly and that's when she really declined. I don't know if she was trying to fit in to his world or just cope, but I'm certain that's around the time she started using heroine. That was the game changer. Once she fell into the heroine hole, she basically surrendered herself to it.

⌐ Colleen: I suspected drug use of some kind, but not heroine.

⌐ Me: I know, me too. Her friend from high school, Kristin, realized it pretty quickly. Her mom is a nurse and they took Rachel to the hospital for an exam. The hospital sent her to detox. I had no idea any of that was happening until Rachel called me one morning and asked me to pick her up from the clinic she was at.

⌐ Colleen: Where was it?

⌐ Me: It is in Charleston. She had some out-patient follow up appointments. Those were in Dunbar. I took her to a couple of them. Then she told me that she felt much better since everything was out of her system and she didn't need to go back. I, being stupid and naïve believed her.

⌐ Colleen: I think it's more that you really wanted that to be true. I mean none of us has any experience with anything like this.

⌐ Me: I don't know. There are only so many ways I can beat myself up about it. All I can say is that if I knew then what I know now, I would have handled it much differently.

DAY 3 – Saturday, September 9, 2017

9:10 am, Conversation with a friend.

↲ Me: I'm starting to figure out how the ICU works. Each nurse is assigned certain patients. They have the same ones for a couple of days then they rotate. Rachel has a new nurse today. I really liked the other one but this one seems good too.

↲ Beth: That's probably a good system. Keeps everything fresh.

↲ Me: True. I have been so impressed with all of them here. They must pick the best nurses for the ICU!

↲ Beth: I admire those that choose that field. It's not an easy job.

↲ Me: It takes a special person with a certain mind set for sure. I've been looking through my phone. Rachel texted me like a week ago on September 1 and asked me to buy her a bike.

↲ Beth: What on earth? Why did she want a bike?

↲ Me: Not sure. She doesn't have her car anymore, maybe she thought it would be easier to get around. I said I would, but before I went to meet her to get it she changed her mind.

↲ Beth: It could have been an impulse thing.

ᒪ Me: Maybe. It's just weird how recently that was. The last text I got from her was just a few days ago on Sept. 4. It says "I love you too momma!"

ᒪ Beth: Wow! That's crazy.

ᒪ Me: Yes. You know she's been struggling for a while, but she ended almost every conversation with I love you. The real Rachel is still in there.

ᒪ Beth: I know.

12:40 pm, Conversation with my daughter.
ᒪ Maddy: Hey so Lollie wants to know if you would like to get some food? She wants to pick u up so u can have a glass of wine.

ᒪ Me: That's sweet! Let me text you in a minute. They just brought Rachel a tray of liquids!

ᒪ Maddy: Okk let me know.

ᒪ Me: She got water!!!

ᒪ Maddy: Yayyyy

ᒪ Me: Now that she got water, she has a new demand! Will you bring her an orange Gatorade?

ᒪ Maddy: Yeaa I will.

ᒪ Me: She did pretty good with her tray. She got water and fruit juice which she guzzled. She got tomato soup that she does not like. And she got a little vanilla ice cream.

ᒪ Maddy: That's good. And that she's awake enough.

⌐Me: Yes. I had to hold the straw or spoon up to her mouth, but she did fine.

⌐Me: Rachel wants to know when you're coming. She wants a Fiji water too!

⌐Maddy: Okkk. Be there in 15

1:52 pm, Conversations between me and 2 friends.
⌐Me: Rachel's sleeping now but she's been pretty restless. Her arm is a little worse. It's more swollen and purple today. Her oxygen level goes down when she pulls the thing out of her nose and her respiration rate keeps going too high. The heart doctor came in to see her and said hopefully Monday for the test if her platelet levels come up from 22 to 50. Other than that just the same stuff. Let the antibiotics do their thing.

⌐Beth: I sure hope so! I'm sure she is quite restless. Still experiencing withdrawal, I imagine.

⌐Me: It's hard to tell what's pain and illness and what's withdrawal. They are giving her meds for both.

⌐Beth: Oh I'm sure! I imagine she's in a lot of pain. The arm alone sounds REALLY painful.

⌐Me: Yes. In the worst spot, infection down to the bone! 😖

⌐Beth: Ohhh… Ugh … hurts my arm just to think about it. I'm sure it looks pretty icky too!

⌐Me: The worst part is bandaged and I have no desire to see it based on the way the better parts look!

⌐ <u>Beth</u>: Oh hell no!!!

2:00 pm

⌐ Nancy: Thanks for the update. Prayers continue…I'll come by tomorrow.

> ⌐ <u>Me</u>: Only if you want to. I don't want anybody to feel like they have to. She will probably be here for a while.

⌐ <u>Nancy</u>: I want to ♥ .

> ⌐ <u>Me</u>: Thanks, Nancy. You're awesome. I don't know how you do it. You sat with us, what about a year and a half ago, when she had to have that abscess drained on her other arm. You must have a strong stomach!

⌐ <u>Nancy</u>: It doesn't bother me…Glad to be there.

2:52 pm, conversation with my sister.

⌐ <u>Colleen</u>: I'll be coming to see you and Rachel tomorrow. Has dad been there? Has Kelly?

> ⌐ <u>Me</u>: Dad and Anna came yesterday. I've been keeping Kelly updated but she hasn't come. I don't want anyone to feel like they have to. There's not much we can do and it's not very pleasant!

⌐ <u>Colleen</u>: I know but I just feel the need to see her even if it's just a few minutes and she doesn't recognize me. I just want to tell her I love her and I also want to see you.

> ⌐ <u>Me</u>: Anyone that wants to come should come. Anyone that doesn't want to or can't shouldn't feel like they have to.

¬ Me: She will recognize you. She was able to talk a little with Dad and Anna. She's out, but if you try to wake her up or start talking to her she responds. I call it semi-conscious. The nurse said somnolent. Anna reminded her about Cubby being her bodyguard when she was a baby. It was like a natural instinct.

¬ Colleen: I remember her laying on a blanket on the floor and him laying close to her watching everyone.

¬ Me: Lol! I wasn't even sure he would let me near her! That's probably why Rachel is such a big animal lover!

¬ Colleen: Lol! Yes, probably! George will probably come tomorrow too.

¬ Me: Sounds good.

7:42 pm
¬ Me: I went to dinner with Maddy and a couple of her friends. It was nice.

¬ Nancy: Are you back at the hospital?

¬ Me: Yes. I worry when I'm not here. I know they'll call if something changes but I don't want Rachel to wake up and me not be here.

¬ Nancy: I totally get it.

⅃ <u>Me</u>: She was kind of in and out today. Kind of fitful. One of the times she tried to wake up she kept saying "I've been a horrible person". I would tell her it was OK and she would say "I love you mommy". I would tell her I loved her too. This was over and over. I feel like she was trying to confess and wanting forgiveness. I pray that God knows what is in her heart.

⅃ <u>Nancy</u>: I know he does…I have no doubt.

DAY 4 – Sunday, September 10, 2017

10:05 am, conversations with 2 friends.

Me: So not as good today. Around 3 a.m. she started having worse respiratory issues and is less coherent. Platelet levels are lower so heart test tomorrow is not looking good. Doctor just came in and they are still talking to hematologist. They are going to do a chest xray to make sure some of the heart growth didn't break off and go to her lungs. They are waiting to get lab work results back to see how to proceed.

Beth: Darn. Do you think her coherency (or lack of it) is partly result of the pain medicines she's getting?

Me: No. The nurse said she gave her pain medicine early this morning after all of this started. Not sure but my guess is to help her breathe deeper. She was in a lot of pain yesterday when she tried to take deep breaths. I know she has the large growth on her heart valves but I worry about infectious fluid in her lungs.

Beth: I guess she has so many issues, can't tell which one to worry about most. Heart, breathing, infection. I never thought of that last one you just said. I really hope they can get the infection under control so they can operate on her heart!! Damn! Wonder what they'll do if that happened?

Me: It's just a wait and see day. I think I'm getting an ulcer. Literally my stomach feels like its bleeding!

⤶ Beth: It certainly is a good possibility. If ever there was a candidate for one, it's you. Might be smart to check it out. You have to take care of yourself, you know. Rachel has several people taking care of her, so think of yourself!!!

⤶ Me: The xray people are already here!

⤶ Beth: Wow! See? She has people taking care of her! And it does sound like she's getting good care.

⤶ Me: She's getting the best care. I don't doubt that at all.

⤶ Me: (sent pic of Rachel) this was Friday when her numbers were better.

⤶ Beth: When her numbers were better? Oh the poor child. So sad.

⤶ Me: You and I see poor child. They see another druggie. I hate that.

⤶ Beth: Sigh...true. But the mother in us knows better.

⤶ Me: Yes. One of the guys who put her catheter in kind of reached out. He said he has a troubled brother so he totally understands that these are people controlled by drugs. It was really nice.

⤶ Beth: If you ever need me to do anything – take dog out, whatever, do not hesitate to let me know.

⤶ Me: Thanks. I appreciate it. It's easier now that Maddy is home.

10:20 am

↲ Nancy: I'll be there a little later. Prayers continue. Have you told Judy?

↳ Me: Thanks. Yes. I have kept her updated.

↲ Nancy: Good. More prayers from Judy and her church. Has Alex kept in contact?

↳ Me: Not really. He knows what's going on but hasn't asked for updates.

↲ Nancy: I know when Halley was sick and Logan was in Morgantown I wanted to keep him from worrying about Halley…sometimes I feel like I did him an injustice. You just don't know what to do.

↳ Me: Unless something changes I'll just wait and give him updates if he asks. He knows the main things. I'm sure in his time he'll ask. I know he's been hurt by the choices she has made. It makes him mad, but they have a bond.

↲ Nancy: So did Halley and Logan.

↳ Me: I remember you telling me that towards the end you would hear them talking during the night. Rachel has always been so proud of Alex and his sports. She didn't like to go to his games, but she was his biggest fan! A few years ago when Alex got in trouble at school and I was freaking out, Rachel wanted to help. She spent the night talking and playing video games with him. It really helped. She really wants to be a good big sister.

↲ Nancy: I know.

↲ Me: Halley had melanoma. It was tragic to lose such an amazing young person who had such a bright future. I feel that way about Rachel. We have been losing her for the last few years, but her illness is addiction. There is a stigma that goes with it. Does that make her less of a person? Does that make me love her any less?

↲ Nancy: Of course not.

↲ Me: To me, loss is loss, pain is pain and love is love...no conditions. Please know that I am not in any way lessening the profound sadness of Halley's story. I still have hope for Rachel. I just don't like the assumed shame of her situation. I think that's what bothers Alex, too.

↲ Nancy: I know.

↲ Me: Thanks, Nancy, for letting me vent.

12:13 pm, conversation with work friend.
↲ Judy: We prayed today at Church and will again this evening.

↲ Me: Thanks! That means a lot!

↲ Judy: BTW yesterday at the grocery store, there was orange Gatorade on almost every aisle!

↲ Me: Lol! Maddy brought her some! She hasn't been awake enough today to ask for anything.

1:12 pm

↲ Me: The chest xray showed fluid in her lungs. She is getting Lasix for that and a unit of blood. They didn't seem like that was unusual so must be par for the course. She's been sleeping all day.

↲ Beth: I'll bet that will help her respiration and breathing. It's good she's sleeping I think. So much easier for her to tolerate pain etc… plus I would think it will help her body heal.

↲ Me: That's what I think too. I'd much rather see her resting than struggling. My niece, Elise, stopped by to see her. She has her masters in nursing and was here checking on some patients. She had on a lab coat. She looked so professional.

↲ Beth: That's nice. I know it helps to have family around.

↲ Me: Definitely. She's such a sweetie. I have also been smiling because I was remembering her bridal shower a few years ago. We played a game that was basically who had the most random thing in their purse. Rachel won. She had a large toenail clipping. It was both disgusting and hilarious!

↲ Beth: LOL! Only Rachel!

5:34 pm
↲ Me: She's been sleeping and mostly unresponsive all day. She got 2 units of blood and Lasix. Her breathing seems a little more stable right now and her numbers look a little better. They may put her on a respirator to give her body a rest from the rapid breathing and let it work on fighting the infection.

꜀ Beth: Now that sounds quite positive!

꜀ Me: She definitely looks more comfortable. Helps me relax a little.

꜀ Nancy: Any changes?

꜀ Me: She got 2 units of blood and the Lasix. She pooped in the bed, got a bath and some pain medicine and is sound asleep again. I'm home. I had things to do here and I think she's going to be out for a while.

꜀ Nancy: Sounds like you left her in a more comfortable condition 🩶

꜀ Me: She looked and sounded better.

8:55 pm, conversation with my sister.
꜀ Colleen: Are you going to the hospital tomorrow or are you going to work?

꜀ Me: I'm going to work. Maddy is going to the hospital. I feel weird about it but right now it's all wait and see. Once we start treatment and surgery that's when I need to be there.

꜀ Colleen: I understand. I can be there during the day when you need me starting after tomorrow. It's important that a family member is there as much as possible.

꜀ Me: I appreciate that. We can talk more tomorrow.

DAY 5, Monday, September 11, 2017

6:56 am, conversation with a friend.
Nancy: How is she this morning?

> Me: I'm still at home. They haven't called so probably the same. Maddy's going this morning.

> Me: I feel so conflicted. I'm so worried I feel like my stomach is bleeding. I've been so consumed with the medical stuff. I have forgotten that her biggest problem is still addiction. When I think about how many times I have gotten my hopes up that she has reached a turning point but was wrong, I get really discouraged. When she could talk she was already asking for her phone and wanting to leave.

Nancy: Well, it's gonna be a battle. Thank God you knew to remove all phone data. She's still going thru withdrawal…is what her pleading says to me. And Maureen, thank God, she's never gotten pregnant!!!!!

> Me: Yes. Withdrawal is one of the biggest battles. The other I think was God's work. If after all of this she wanted to go back to that lifestyle, I don't think I could bare it.

Nancy: Let's focus on her health right now…God will work in this.

> Me: You're right, of course.

11:20 am, conversation with my daughter.
> Me: Does Rachel know you're there?

⌐ Maddy: I mean I told her and I tried to give her some water but when I put the straw in her mouth she fell back asleep.

⌐ Maddy: And she has some crud on her tongue, it looks like there's a little orange pill on the tip of her tongue but it's just dryness.

> ⌐ Me: She has had that crud. The nurse tried to clean her mouth with a toothbrush but she said it kind of made it worse. I have no idea what that junk is!

⌐ Maddy: No wonder she wanted water. I bet her mouth tastes terrible!

> ⌐ Me: You're a good sister to be there taking care of her.

⌐ Maddy: I want to. She would do it for me.

> ⌐ Me: She definitely would. She always wants to be there for you. Remember a couple of years ago when you were driving home from Morgantown in the snow. You were so scared. She stayed on the phone with you almost the whole time talking you through it.

⌐ Maddy: Yes, I remember that. She made me laugh and think about other things.

> ⌐ Me: The time that has really stayed with me was your birthday before last. She was such a mess with her teeth and things, but she would not miss your birthday. She showed up that night with a little basket of gifts. She didn't stay long. I think she just wanted you to know she remembered. It touched me.

ᒾ Maddy: Stop mom. You're going to make me cry.

ᒾ Me: Sorry. Not trying to.

11:31 am, conversation between me and a friend.
ᒾ Me: Here's Maddy's update: Her respiratory level is steady at 26, she said it raised a little to 35 but that's still good and they think the platelet levels are back down to 20 and she's still only waking up for like 30 seconds at a time.

ᒾ Beth: That sounds promising. Is 26 a good respiratory level? Is 35 better? How is Maddy doing?

ᒾ Me: 26 is great! It's supposed to be between 12 and 20. Maddy just got there. She slept through her alarm! She's doing OK. Hanging in there.

ᒾ Beth: I'm sure it's somewhat overwhelming for her.

ᒾ Me: Yes, definitely. It shocks me to think how much she has seen. She's been surrounded by this stuff for a while. She has multiple friends that have had addiction issues and now seeing her sister like this. I'm so thankful that she has had the strength to make better choices.

ᒾ Beth: Maybe seeing what drugs have done to people she cares about has had a big impact. Hard lesson to learn, but I bet she has.

ᒾ Me: You're right. I don't see how it couldn't have an impact.

1:30 pm
ᒾ Maddy: They are hoping to try the TEE at the end of the week.

⤶ Me: They were originally going to try to do it today.

⤶ Maddy: I told Gaby about it and she is gonna come by when she gets off work, I asked her what time that was so maybe she could come in with you.

⤶ Me: Ok. I should be there around 5.

⤶ Maddy: She said she's gonna be here about 4:30 and Judy's pastor just came by and said a prayer for Rachel and it was super sweet! He gave me his card and said if we ever need anything or if we have an update just to call him!

⤶ Me: Wow! I have tears in my eyes!

⤶ Maddy: Yeaa it gave me chills. The good chills though. Lol.

⤶ Me: I bet!

2:10 pm, conversation with 2 friends.
⤶ Me: TEE heart test put off until the end of the week. Judy's pastor was just there and said a prayer for Rachel!

⤶ Beth: Bad about heart test. But that's so nice that the pastor came by.

⤶ Me: I know. I teared up when Maddy told me!

⤶ Nancy: Prayers.🙏 I was just sitting here thinking about her. 🩶

4:54 pm

⅃ Me: Just got here. She's on a bigger respirator than just the oxygen they had her on. The platelet numbers are better. She's at 31 needs to be at 50 for heart test. She's been out most of the day. Her arm though. Wow! It looks awful. It's extremely swollen and kind of purple.

⅃ Beth: Sounds like maybe we are on right track. Hopefully platelets will be up to 50 by the end of the week. The arm! Ick. I'm sure it's icky and quite painful. When are they going to operate on it?

⅃ Me: I don't know. If they can't do a heart test because of bleeding risks I'm guessing the arm surgery may not happen for a while.

⅃ Beth: True.

⅃ Me: I'm getting a medical education. The low platelets mean her blood won't clot properly and she's a bleeding risk. I'll confide in you. I'm terrified she's going to lose her arm.

⅃ Beth: I didn't want to come right out and say it but that's why I asked when they can operate. Let's pray not!!!!!

⅃ Me: Also her heart condition is called endocarditis. I had never heard of it. I guess it can happen for many reasons but is a risk factor to addicts.

⅃ Beth: We are both learning things!

⌐ Me: I feel stupid. I should have been more aware of things. I knew she could overdose. I knew she could get a tainted drug and I knew about withdrawal. I did not know about all of this other medical stuff. It was too easy to assume it must be withdrawal if she didn't feel good. I didn't know to look for all this other stuff. Maybe I could have talked her into a medical check-up even if she didn't want rehab. I could have tried to scare her with it and make her think!

⌐ Beth: There is no way you could have known. How could you?

⌐ Me: I mean they don't talk about this kind of stuff on the news, but I'm her mom. I feel like I should have been able to tell something wasn't right.

⌐ Beth: Come on. Are you psychic now?! She wasn't living with you. When was the last time you saw her?

⌐ Me: We have talked and texted, but I haven't seen her since June. She didn't look good, but she hasn't looked like herself for a while. I talked to her on the phone a couple of weeks ago and she told me she wasn't feeling good. I asked her if she was withdrawing. She said no and went into this story about how a girl wanted to beat her up because of someone that "serves" them. I said I didn't want to hear about that and hung up. Why didn't I talk to her more? I feel so guilty.

⌐ Beth: Stop that. You and I both know she more than likely would not have accepted any form of treatment. She is an adult and if she needed a doctor she should have told you. Then the texts about the bike, no indication that she was sick.

↲ Me: I guess, but I'm having a really hard time with that. Sometimes I would get so angry and frustrated with her. She has stolen from me and lied to me. We have had some big fights, but I never wanted to be so hard core that I gave her ultimatums or kicked her out. Everyone was telling me that I had to be tough and that she had to hit rock bottom. I tried, but that's just not me. And I'm not sure there is a rock bottom for opioid addicts. It's more like they have to be freed from a captor. I have never really known how to handle any of this or what to do.

7:42 pm, conversation with my sister.
↲ Colleen: I'm so appreciative of your updates. It brought tears to my eyes to hear that Judy and one of the pastors came to the hospital to pray for Rachel. She will be getting a lot of true prayers from some of the best Christians I've ever known. I can only imagine how difficult it is for you to see her like this. What time will you get there tomorrow?

↲ Me: I am so grateful for the prayers! Maddy will be here during the day. I will get here around 4:45. Kim and Gaby came to see her today.

↲ Colleen: That's nice. How was it?

↲ Me: It was really good. I was starting to freak out a little so it was nice to see them. I haven't talked to either one of them in a while. Gaby is teaching now, all grown up! And Kim understands a lot more of the medical stuff than I do.

↲ Colleen: What did she say?

꜀ Me: She had never heard of some of the stuff either! She was able to explain to me what all of the numbers on the machines are.

꜀ Colleen: Did Rachel know they were there?

꜀ Me: I didn't think so, she never opened her eyes. But before they left, she smiled at them! I hope she could hear us. We told a lot of funny stories about her! You know how she likes that!

꜀ Colleen: I guess I didn't realize that she and Gaby were that close.

꜀ Me: Oh yes. When she was little she hung out more with the other cousins but she and Gaby went to high school together. That's what Gaby was talking about. They thought they were so cool running around together. She was just telling me about some of the funny situations they got in to. They also had an annual tradition of going shopping the day after Christmas. Granny always gave them money so of course they had to spend it immediately. Gaby said they always had so much fun.

꜀ Colleen: I can imagine, giggling teenagers.

꜀ Me: Exactly. Kim was telling me about a time when Rachel was little and was with them so often. They went to visit Kim's parents. Before they left Kim's mom told Kim's kids to give meemaw and pawpaw hugs and kisses before they left. Rachel got in line with her cousins for hugs and kisses too!

꜀ Colleen: Awe. So cute!

꜀ Me: Yes. It was nice to take a break from the stress and laugh a little.

DAY 6, Tuesday, September 12, 2017

8:36 am, conversation with my sister.

↲ Me: I stopped by to see Rachel this morning. Maddy will be going over again today and I'll go back after work. She was breathing on her own and the numbers looked great. She woke up and talked a little and drank a lot of water! The arm is still really swollen but she appeared pretty good.

↲ Kelly: That's great. So good to hear some good news.

↲ Me: I know. It's been so freaky. I was telling Colleen the other night, everything's being thrown at us so quickly. I'm kind of numb, just trying to take it all in.

↲ Kelly: Yes and I'm not sure what to do. Just waiting makes me feel helpless.

↲ Me: Don't I know it. I'm not even sure how to react to things. What's normal? What's not? What does it all mean? She's coherent one moment then not the next. Hard to make any sense from it.

↲ Kelly: I don't think we can right now. That's the hardest part.

↲ Me: I don't think that Rachel even knows how sick she is. The other day, she kept asking me if she could borrow $2. She said she was going to walk to the store and get a Gatorade. I told her she was too sick to go to the store. She kept saying "I'm not that sick". Silly girl. You know how stubborn she can be once she gets an idea in her head!

↲ Kelly: Yes I do! And I know how silly she can be. She can always make me laugh.

↲ Me: She is funny. It's always the random things that she does or says that crack me up. Or the influence of a bad uncle! Remember when Scott took her to Kings Island?

↲ Kelly: OMG! I know what you're going to say. The epic farting contest?!!!

↲ Me: Lol! Yes. They should not have been allowed to travel together!

8:45 am, conversation with a friend.
↲ Me: Rachel is breathing on her own this morning!

↲ Nancy: Wonderful! So, no respirator?

↲ Me: Not this morning and her respiration numbers were excellent!

↲ Nancy: What a relief!

↲ Me: I know. I was so freaked out last night I had to see her this morning for peace of mind.

↲ Nancy: I was too…and I didn't even "see" her on the respirator.

↲ Me: I don't think it was a full-fledged respirator, it was just a bigger machine than the oxygen she had been on. But I'm glad it's gone!

3:16 pm, simultaneous conversations with 2 friends.

⌐ Me: I'm at the hospital now. Maddy has a sore throat and decided not to come today. I just got to talk to the kidney doctor that I just found out she had. I didn't realize he had been treating her because her kidneys were not working when she got here. He said he is supplementing her potassium but she looks better than when she first got here. So that's good!

⌐ Beth: Everything looks like it's going in the right direction today! Hallelujah!

⌐ Nancy: Yes, it is good. If all of her organs were infected…I can see why the kidneys weren't working. Anybody mention her liver?

⌐ Me: Yes, they are watching it. They know she has Hep B and C.

⌐ Nancy: Ok. Good. I'm glad things look better today.

⌐ Me: She's definitely more responsive and talking more! Her arm looks a little better today too.

⌐ Beth: Oh good!

⌐ Me: The nurse told me that Rachel has been talking to her all day. She was able to tell her that she is the oldest with a sister and a brother. She told the nurse that she wanted a Coke. They made a deal that if Rachel ate her chicken noodle soup she would get it for her. I'm glad she's having a good day, but I hate that I missed most of it.

⌐ Beth: You're there now. Enjoy it.

٦ Me: I am, but the guilt! The nurse said Rachel remembered I was there this morning and asked her where I was!

٦ Me: Something just happened. She had an episode or something. She started babbling and her eyes lost focus. They shined a light in them and said her pupils were uneven. Not sure what they're going to do. It's either withdrawal or a brain bleed.

٦ Beth: Oh no!!! I sure pray it's withdraw!!! Let me know ASAP.

٦ Me: It was really creepy. She was doing well then all of a sudden just this weird repetitive babble.

٦ Me: She only got one question right. They asked her what her sister's name was and she bellowed "Madeline Lewis". The rest was just repetitive sounds.

٦ Nancy: Oh, my lord...prayers lifting

٦ Me: They are taking her for a CT scan of her head and stomach.

7:03 pm

↲ Me: So no brain bleed and no new strokes. She is having a really bad evening. Kind of took a turn for the worse. Found out she has 2 strains of infection. MRSA and another that I can't pronounce, selatia or serratia. Both are very hard to treat. She has a fever and seems to be in a lot of pain. Doctor said she could be "decomposing". The heart valve could be getting overwhelmed with infection. He said they will fight as hard as they can for her and keep her comfortable. Then they will decide what else can be done.

↲ Me: They're putting her on life support. They are not giving up just precautionary.

↲ Beth: Decomposing????? That's the word he used? Does that mean what it sounds like? I'm sure she is in pain. At least no brain bleed! Whew. And it sounds like she is getting great care. I just wish they could get her to the point where they could operate and do other stuff they need to. But I guess I need to be patient. It's a long process.

↲ Me: He actually said decomposing. That's a horrible word. I'm hoping it means something different in medical terms than what it normally would. I'm every bit as impatient as you. It's heart wrenching to see her in pain. I'm getting so frustrated just waiting!

↲ Nancy: I'm so sorry…prayers continue 🙏

↲ Me: It's gruesome. It's like she is wrestling with demons. She's moaning and babbling and crying out. Her eyes are totally out there. They're open but she's not there. I had to step out while they clean her up.

↲ Beth: Oh poor, poor girl! I don't know what withdrawal is like but it sounds like that's what it is. But probably made worse by the other pain she's in.

↲ Beth: and Life support!!! What the...?? What does all this mean??? I'm freaking out. But just precautionary?

↲ Me: Because she's struggling so much they think it will help her body rest and keep her airways open.

↲ Beth: Oh ok. That relieves me somewhat.

↲ Me: They've been brutally honest with me. They can't guarantee anything. "Some make it. Some don't". But we know how stubborn and sassy Rachel is. They don't!

↲ Beth: True that!!! She's saying...

8:11 pm, message to my son, Rachel's brother.
↲ Me: I need to let you know what's going on. Rachel was stable but took a turn for the worse this evening. They are putting her on life support. Not giving up. Just precautionary.

No response

8:21 pm, conversation with my sister.

⌐ Kelly: I'm sad to hear she's not doing well this evening. But you never know what tomorrow will bring. It sounds like it's going to be a long road of ups and downs. Hopefully more ups. I don't want to sound corny but you are one of the strongest people I know and I really admire that. Love you so much.

    ⌐ Me: I don't feel strong at all. I feel sick and numb. My stomach is in knots. I can see and hear what's happening but I can't comprehend it.

    8:24 pm, conversation with my sister-in-law.
    ⌐ Me: Rachel is having a rough day. They made the decision to put her on life support for precautionary reasons.

⌐ Kim: Oh gosh I'm so sorry! When you say life support, do you mean a ventilator?

    ⌐ Me: They said life support. I have no clue what that means.

⌐ Kim: Ok, is there anything we can do for you? Tom and I will stop in tomorrow and check on her if that's ok.

    ⌐ Me: I haven't seen her yet but the nurse just came out and said she did great. I'm relieved! Absolutely you all can come any time. I plan on being here most of the day. I want to talk to the doctors. Not that I will understand what they say. I'll tell you and you can interpret for me!

⌐ Kim: Ok sounds good. We'll see you tomorrow then. Please call at any time if you need us.

    8:25 pm, conversation with my sister.

⤸ <u>Colleen</u>: Kelly told me what's going on. We're on our way there.

⤸ <u>Me</u>: No need. It's more precautionary. I'm just waiting to check on her after they hook her up. I want to see her then I'm going home.

⤸ <u>Colleen</u>: We're already here.

Colleen, George and I held hands and prayed by Rachel's bedside.

DAY 7, Wednesday, September 13, 2017

9:33 am, conversation with a friend.
⌐ Me: Kind of scary. She wasn't here when I first walked in, but she's back in the room now. She was having some testing including an MRI. The doctor is going to look at it. The CT scan on the abdomen shows infection in her liver and spleen. Arm looks a little better. She's hanging in there!

⌐ Beth: Is she still on life support? Or have they taken her off?

⌐ Me: She's still on it and they are going to do tube feedings. The doctor said they will start to slowly bring her out of sedation and see how she does. He talked about possibly removing breathing tube in a couple days.

⌐ Beth: Now that sounds somewhat promising! Hopefully she'll breathe easy on her own when they do.

⌐ Me: Yes. I think she's getting a really good rest right now.

⌐ Beth: Which is something she really needs.

⌐ Me: Absolutely. It's the best thing for her.

⌐ Me: Rachel has a new nurse today. It's a guy that she went to school with. They've known each other since kindergarten. They played soccer together when they were little. I didn't even recognize him at first!

⌐ Beth: It's a small world.

꜀ Me: And they graduated with the nurse practitioner. Both the nurse and nurse practitioner said this is the first time they have taken care of a classmate. It's kind of weird but mostly good, because I know they truly care about Rachel!

꜀ Beth: That's great.

10:59 am, message to group.
꜀ Me: The nurse practitioner just sat me down and gave me the reality of the situation. The MRI showed pieces of the infectious growth on her heart went to her brain. It was explained to me that the growth is very large and is now breaking off and traveling in her blood. The only option is an extremely high-risk surgery to remove the growth and replace the valve. She is not a good candidate to survive surgery. Without surgery the growth is going to keep breaking off and overwhelming her body. The nurse practitioner knows Rachel and is fighting to give her a chance with the surgery if anyone will take her as a patient with her illness and her history.

⌐ Beth: Well, here's my thoughts and, of course, I'm definitely no medical professional-farthest thing from it- but it sounds to me if she doesn't have the surgery, that growth will keep breaking up and eventually kill her. I mean, if it already went to her brain, that's serious! I'll bet that's why she was acting crazy yesterday. And if she does have the surgery, she MIGHT die. Yes, it's risky but it sounds like she at least has a chance if they operate but if they don't, she doesn't. It's all so overwhelming to me. I can't imagine how it must be to you. They keep coming up with something new that is wrong. Seems like every time you give me positive news, at least two other pieces of bad news follow. So many questions! Like is that piece still in her brain? Would they operate on that? Are the antibiotics working to get the infection down? Do they know how long they can wait to see if she gets strong enough to operate? Etc…see what I mean? Even I am overwhelmed!!

⌐ Beth: And seriously honestly! How are you holding up? What can I do? I feel helpless. And how are Maddy and Alex handling all this?

⌐ Me: There are several places on her brain like embolisms. I understand things the same way you do. A chance with surgery or certain death without. I still maintain they are underestimating how strong willed and determined she is. That will serve her well. Maddy's kind of freaking out. I told Alex last night and have gotten no response. I'm somewhat sleep deprived and go between uncontrollable tears and exhausted numb. That's my baby girl. I can't put it in words.

⌐ Nancy: It's all in God's hands now. 🙏 Things sound so grim. Are you at the hospital now?

↲ Me: Yes

↲ Nancy: I just sent my church an update to continue to pray about. I love you and your family, Maureen.

↲ Me: Thanks Nancy. I love you too.

11:07 am, conversation with my daughter.
↲ Me: Are you coming today?

↲ Maddy: Idkk. I want to! But it's kinda been messing with my head like giving me anxiety when I go there…

↲ Me: I get it. Come if you want to. I hate to think this way but will you have regrets if you don't? I'm not giving up. You know how strong willed and determined Rachel is. That will help her.

↲ Maddy: I just don't think I can right now. Maybe later.

↲ Me: I understand. Try to think good thoughts and be positive. Also, will you try to call Alex? I sent him a text but he hasn't responded.

↲ Maddy: Okk. I will.

11:11 am, conversation with my sister.
↲ Kelly: God I hope someone will give her the chance. As scary as the surgery sounds at least it's something.

↲ Me: I know. It's just waiting which is excruciating. I feel like I'm going to burst and then I cry.

ᒧ Kelly: I can't imagine. Just hearing about it is hard enough, being there must be so intense.

> ᒧ Me: It is. She's just lying there with all those wires and machines. You saw all that the other day. Now I can't even see her face anymore with the breathing tube. I find myself just staring at all of the numbers and lines.

ᒧ Kelly: I'll be praying. Let me know if you need anything.

> ᒧ Me: I will. Thanks.

1:37 pm, response of my son from yesterday's message.
ᒧ Alex: What r her chances?

> ᒧ Me: The heart surgeon just said that with surgery she has a chance. They are transferring her to Memorial ASAP. The surgery won't be for a little while. You should try to have a great birthday weekend and maybe come in once the surgery is scheduled. I'll let you know if anything changes.

> *4:37 pm, message to group.*
> ᒧ Me: Prayer is working. A surgeon at Memorial agreed to take her. She will be transferred there ASAP. He was very clear that without surgery she has 0 chance of survival. With surgery she has a small chance but it's extremely high risk. I'll take it! Challenge accepted! He doesn't know Rachel like we do!

Conversation with a friend.
ᒧ Beth: TRUE! I feel so smart! I said what the doctor said. Any idea when they'll do it?

⌐ Me: Smart … smart ass, whatever! Lol! They will have to wait a couple weeks because of the infection spots on her brain. They will monitor her closely because he doesn't want it to turn into an emergency surgery.

⌐ Beth: 😁 Ha ha! You're so funny! As much as I was hoping more like tomorrow (patience never was one of my virtues) I guess two weeks will give her time to fight more and get stronger. Less infection!!

⌐ Me: That's my hope too. I'm just so happy to have a plan and be taking some kind of action. Just sitting here waiting was really getting to me.

⌐ Beth: Yeah. At least having a plan makes you feel in control.

⌐ Me: You are right! And Memorial is the best for heart surgery. I really like the doctor. He spoke in a way that I could understand. He actually said that he will be treating her symptoms, her real illness is the brain disease of addiction. He really got it.

⌐ Beth: Yes, he did. That's great. Good surgeon at a good hospital. They are ranked way up there nationally.

⌐ Me: We are just waiting for a bed to open up in one of the 3 ICUs. I know it will happen once I leave tonight!

Conversation with a friend.
⌐ Nancy: I had sent my church an update today. My Pastor sent me a text that faith as small as mustard seed…

꜀ Me: Yes. I agree with that!

Conversation with my sister-in-law.
꜀ Kim: OK, thanks for the update. Let us know what unit she's in please. Always know we will have you all in our prayers.

꜀ Me: I know. I will. Thanks!

Conversation with work friend.
꜀ Judy: WOW. Who is the surgeon?

꜀ Me: I can't remember. I'll find out. I'm so happy at the moment. We found a surgeon who will do it and he gave me a little hope.

꜀ Judy: I'm so glad. A little hope can mean so much!

6:20 pm, message to group.
꜀ Me: She will be in the CPICU in the new part of Memorial, 5th floor, bed 16.

꜀ Beth: Wow! They really are moving on this.

꜀ Me: They want her there in case an emergency happens. They have the right equipment there.

꜀ Nancy: Cardio Pulmonary Intensive Care Unit. New…is good.

꜀ Me: Yes. That's right. We are just waiting for the ambulance. She's moving tonight. It's in the new unit. It's supposed to be really nice and much more comfortable for the visitors!

꜀ Nancy: 🖤🙏

╛ Me: I want to go check on her once she's there but then I want to sleep! I think I'll be able to rest tonight. I have a good feeling about things. A much better feeling than I had last night.

╛ Kim: OK thanks for the info. Did she make the move ok?

╛ Me: They are just moving her now. They said it will be a couple of hours before I can see her. It was pretty involved just to get her ready to move. It took a long time to unhook things and get her set back up on mobile equipment. They were so careful and thorough. The nurse helped them. It was impressive how they all worked together.

╛ Kim: I bet. That's good to hear.

╛ Me: Just letting you know, the nurse at Memorial just called. Rachel is there and stable.

╛ Kelly: That's great. Thanks for the update. Are you going to see her tonight?

╛ Me: I was going to, but I'm so tired. The nurse assured me she would call if anything changes, so I think I'll wait until tomorrow.

╛ Kelly: Good plan. Try to get some rest.

╛ Me: I will. Good night.

DAY 8, Thursday, September 14, 2017

10:21 am, conversation with my sister.

↲ <u>Colleen</u>: I'm soooo sorry I didn't get back to you yesterday. I'm glad you feel a little better with Rachel being at Memorial and the Dr. agreeing to do the surgery in 2 weeks. I know it's an uphill battle but our Rachel is one stubborn girl! Kelly told me that Dad and Anna were there and then Tom and Kim. Was Kim helpful? I always thought she was so nice.

↲ <u>Me</u>: I'm at work this morning trying to stay caught up. I'm going to the hospital this afternoon. Kim was very helpful. She understands more medical stuff than I do and she's not afraid to ask questions!

11:19 am, conversation with 2 friends.

↲ <u>Beth</u>: I'm assuming no news is good news.

↲ <u>Me</u>: She was transferred to Memorial late last night. They called me and told me she was there and was stable. I waited until the ambulance got there for her last night. They said it would be a couple hours before I could see her and it was so late I went home. I missed work Tuesday afternoon and all day yesterday. I'm at the office now trying to get caught up so I haven't seen her. I'm going over this afternoon.

↲ <u>Beth</u>: Ok. Keep me posted.

↲ <u>Nancy</u>: That's good news!

↲ <u>Me</u>: Yes. I'm glad she's there with all of the right equipment for her!

2:02 pm, conversation with a friend.
⅃ <u>Me</u>: I finally found her! It's a really nice room. There is a reclining couch, 2 chairs and 2 TVs' plus her own bathroom. She appears pretty good. Still sedated and on the ventilator. I haven't talked to anyone yet.

⅃ <u>Beth</u>: Sounds nice! I think I'll move in! Lol

⅃ <u>Me</u>: I know. It's clean and peaceful! And no animals jumping on me when I walked in! Rachel's animals I might add!

⅃ <u>Beth</u>: I know Zeppelin. There's also a cat right?

⅃ <u>Me</u>: 2 cats! Honestly every time she is away from home and gets homesick, she gets a pet. Somehow I always end up taking care of them!

⅃ <u>Beth</u>: That's right. I know about the calico kitten. The other one came back from New Jersey with her right?

⅃ <u>Me</u>: Yes. That's the one that I had to pick up at the police station in PA.

⅃ <u>Beth</u>: What?! When was this?

⅃ <u>Me</u>: This was right before she went to the rehab in FL a couple of years ago. I think you were on your cruise. Did I not tell you about this? She called me hysterical one morning while I was getting ready for work. She was telling me some horrible things that were happening where she was staying in NJ.

⅃ <u>Beth</u>: I never really understood how she ended up in NJ to begin with! I was glad when she came back and was ready for rehab.

↲ Me: Me too, but if I had known how bad she was I would have tried to make arrangements to go get her or fly her back or something.

↲ Beth: What happened?

↲ Me: She was hysterical and saying she needed to leave, so I said come on. I had no idea that she was just going to leave from wherever she was right then. She had her kitten with her and that's about all and she just left. No directions, none of her belongings, nothing.

↲ Beth: OMG. Not good.

↲ Me: No. I heard from her on the trip for a while then nothing. It was getting late and she should have made it home and I hadn't heard from her in a while. Finally, she called and was not making any sense. She said she was driving in and out of traffic like she was on a racetrack. She said she wrecked her car, but someone showed up and already fixed it. Then she said she was lost and she was scared. I was freaking out.

↲ Beth: No doubt. How did you find her?

↲ Me: I was able to get her to describe her surroundings. She had also been talking to her friend Kristin. She and I figured out she was in PA and called the police. When they found her she was just sitting in her car on the side of the road and had been there for a few hours. All of the things she was telling me were just hallucinations or something.

↲ Beth: Wow! It's a wonder she wasn't in a wreck.

↲ Me: I know. It makes me cringe to think about it. They took her to a hospital, took the kitten to the station and had her car towed. I know now that she was withdrawing from heroine and Xanax. If I had known before she left, I would have tried to talk her out of driving. It could have been catastrophic. I swear I think Brad must have been watching over her.

↲ Beth: How did you get her car back?

↲ Me: My brother in law went with me that night. He drove her car back and I brought her and the kitten home the next morning.

↲ Beth: I can't believe I didn't know this. That's wild. That was so nice of your brother in law.

↲ Me: Yes it was. I am very thankful!

3:38 pm, conversation with my daughter.
↲ Me: Rachel is in a really nice room. You'll like it a lot better here. You don't have to get buzzed back in every time you leave. That's nice.

↲ Maddy: Lol! Good! How's Rachel?

↲ Me: About the same. She's still sedated so I can't try to talk to her. I'm just sitting here watching her. It's making me wonder if she is dreaming. Like what thought processes she has in this state.

↲ Maddy: Yeah. Idk.

6:07 pm

⌐ Me: It's definitely more comfortable here. She's about the same today. They tried to start bringing her out of sedation but it didn't go well so she's fully sedated again. She also hasn't been able to tolerate the tube feedings. Every time they try she chokes and starts to vomit. The nurse is having them check out her stomach. A bunch of alarms go off when that happens and they have to suction her. It's creepy.

⌐ Me: I'm starting to feel down again. I got excited when they moved her and a surgeon was talking about her surgery but then reality comes back and I realize how far she has to go.

⌐ Beth: Is she still on life support?

⌐ Me: Yes. The original plan was to slowly bring her out of sedation and hopefully off of the ventilator. The surgeon said that would be a factor in when they can do surgery but as of today, it's not going well. I guess they will try again tomorrow. She also has a persistent fever that keeps coming back.

⌐ Beth: I wish they could do the heart surgery sooner. I know it's not the answer to everything but I think it's a big thing.

⌐ Me: If it's done too soon the new valve could get infected.

⌐ Beth: Ohhh…boy am I getting a medical education! I feel like I could be a doctor and skip med school.

7:38 pm
⌐ Me: I played "The Devil Went Down to Georgia" for Rachel. I think she liked it.

⌐ Beth: Fantastic Idea! I'm sure she can hear it. I've heard it said people who are sedated and even comatose can hear what's going on around them.

⌐ Beth: I read a story about a woman in the hospital who was comatose. Her greedy children were there discussing the inheritance they were going to get. No concern for their mother. She woke up! Wrote them all out of the will! She lived another year! Lol

⌐ Me: Lol. I love it! I need to get Maddy here to play her favorite songs. I know some from dancing and some classic rock. Maddy knows which rap songs she likes.

⌐ Beth: I don't listen to much rap.

⌐ Me: I don't either. Rachel has always been a huge fan. She loves the beats. I asked her once why she listens to rap. I said it has no melody. She said the rhythms...its art. Could be why she loved dancing so much, especially tap.

⌐ Beth: She danced for a long time didn't she?

⌐ Me: Yes. Since she was 3. She always loved it. I could use it as leverage! Like if she didn't do a chore I could say no dance class if you don't get it done! You know us moms use what we can!

⌐ Beth: 😄 True!

↓ Me: Those dance competitions were so much fun. I miss it. It seems like a lifetime ago. She was so beautiful on stage with those long legs! And I could always see how much she loved it by the look of joy on her face.

↓ Beth: I remember. Back then we were either at gymnastics meets with Samantha and Maddy or dance competitions with Jessica and Rachel. Good times!

↓ Me: Very good times. I started to watch an old recital video the other night. It was before one of Rachel's dances. The stage was dark. You could hear her friends yelling for her "Go Rachel". They were all so supportive of each other.

↓ Beth: Oh yes, very positive. It was good for self-esteem.

↓ Me: And it helped Rachel work out some of her anxiety. The big toe on each of her feet arch up. She and her dance teacher thought it allowed her to get extra sounds from her tap shoes. Her dance teacher was awesome. She was someone Rachel could talk to. It made her feel special. It was just such a good thing to be part of. I'm really grateful she had that.

↓ Beth: There are a lot more benefits than just learning dances.

↓ Me: I agree. I still have all of her recital costumes. I keep them stored for her kids one day. I know how much she always loved to dress up. I thought it would be cool for her kids to have the costume and a picture of her wearing it.

↓ Beth: Great idea!

7:54 pm, conversation with my sister-in-law.

ᒣ Kim: How's Rachel doing?

> ᒣ Me: She's about the same I think. Her fever keeps coming back. They think she has another abscess on her forearm that may be an active source of infection. They were going to try to bring her out of sedation but that's not going well. She is not able to tolerate the tube feedings. Every time they try she starts to vomit and choke which sets off a bunch of alarms and they have to suction her. I don't know if that's normal.

ᒣ Kim: I don't either. So are they trying to wean her from the ventilator? Bring out of sedation?

> ᒣ Me: They were trying to slowly cut back on the medicine keeping her sedated and then try to get her off of the ventilator. When they try her heart rate goes up and she gets really restless and starts the weird breathing.

ᒣ Kim: Oh ok gotcha. Would it be ok if I come down there around 8-8:30 in the morning and stay an hour or so?

> ᒣ Me: That would be great. I won't be here in the morning. Maddy is supposed to be at some point. Feel free to ask them any questions. Just let me know what you find out!

ᒣ Kim: Ok thanks. I sure will!

8:40 pm
ᒣ Nancy: Thinking of you, my bible class prayed for you both this evening 🙏

꜏ Me: Thanks! Add Tim and Rick to your list. I saw Tim here at the hospital. They are flying Rick to Cleveland tonight by helicopter.

꜏ Nancy: Gee, that's terrible…yes, I'll keep them in prayer too.

꜏ Me: It was so weird. I was just sitting in Rachel's room and I could hear a man talking to the nurse outside. I looked up and it was Tim. I haven't seen him in months. It's a very strange place to cross paths!

꜏ Nancy: Is he OK? Was he upset?

꜏ Me: He is doing OK. He was definitely worried. He didn't know about Rachel. I told him what was going on. He told me about Rick. We hugged. There was just an understanding that we didn't really have to say anything about. It was comforting for me. I hope it was for him too.

DAY 9, Friday, September 15, 2017

8:13 am, conversation with my sister-in-law.
↲ Kim: I'm with Rachel. The nurse says she's
about the same. Hemoglobin went up. Platelets
have dropped a little but he said she shouldn't
need blood today. She's resting comfortably.

↲ Me: That's good. Thanks!

1:30 pm, conversation with a friend.
↲ Me: I feel so torn. I want to be at the hospital
with Rachel, but I also want to save my time so I
can be off more after her surgery.

↲ Nancy: I know it's tough but try not to worry
about it. Rachel is sedated right now so there's
not much you can do. She will need you more
when she's more coherent. You have other
things to worry about right now!

↲ Me: You're right. I feel guilty not being there,
but I will be glad to have the time with her when
she needs me more. Plus, it's Friday. I can be at
the hospital all weekend.

↲ Nancy: They will call you if anything changes.

↲ Me: Yes. Thanks!

4:28 pm, conversation with my niece.
↲ Gaby: Hey… Just wanted to check and see
how Rach is doing. I haven't heard back from
Maddy so I thought I'd ask you.

↲ Me: Not much change. I'm heading over there
now. Maddy did tell you she was transferred to
Memorial right?

↳ Gaby: She didn't. Glad to know that though. I am going to come to see her tomorrow. She's been on my heart of course.

↳ Me: I know.

5:10 pm, message to group.
↳ Me: Rachel's platelets came up enough to do the TEE test this evening. Then they will know exactly what kind of surgery she has to have.

Conversation with a friend.
↳ Beth: Well now that IS great news. I had to look up TEE test. My, the education I'm getting. When are they going to do it?

↳ Me: Around 6. I don't know when I'll know what they find but I'm happy with forward progress. They also had the stroke doctor come and check her. He said as of right now she's safe for surgery. He said the bigger issue for her currently is the heart. So that's good too. I think they may try to do surgery soon before she has a larger stroke.

↳ Beth: 🙂 Sounds like it!!

Response from my sister-in-law.
↳ Kim: Yes, that's good news. Thanks for the update.

Conversation with a friend.
↳ Nancy: Thank the Lord! I'm so happy! Rosemary is praying for both of you too 🙏

↳ Me: Thanks!

↳ Nancy: I'll be up tomorrow.

˄ Me: Ok. That sounds great! Maybe we will know more by then. I'll let you know when I find out the results of the test tonight.

˄ Nancy: Send the message at any hour!

˄ Me: Ok.

˄ Nancy: Every time I wake up at night I pray for you, Rachel, medical staff and your family.

˄ Me: You're the best! I think it's helping!

6:14 pm, message to group.
˄ Me: The doctor said she does this test about 6 times a week and she has not seen a growth that large in about 4 years. She said Rachel needs surgery soon. She also thinks there may be another infection in one of the ventricles or something like that. That's all I know right now.

Conversation with work friend.
˄ Judy: Oh my. You knew it was bad. Did she give any indication of how soon?

˄ Me: No. But she let me see some of the procedure. The growth looked like a wing fluttering up and down with her heart beat. I think the biggest risk is bigger chunks of it breaking loose and going to her brain or lungs or something. Smaller pieces are already breaking off.

Conversation with a friend.
˄ Beth: Wild! They certainly move fast. What causes such a thing? Since it's so big, I wonder how long it's been growing.

⅃ Me: The doctor said those things grow really slowly. She must have been very sick for a while.

Conversation with a friend.
⅃ Nancy: We'll just pray the antibiotics do their thing ASAP!!

⅃ Me: She let me see some of the procedure. The growth looked kind of like a wing that fluttered up and down with her heart beat. But like a moth wing, kind of thin.

⅃ Nancy: What a description!

⅃ Me: Do you like my expert medical terms?!

⅃ Nancy: Yep…my imagination went wild! ... but nothing "medical" about it.

Response from my sister.
⅃ Kelly: God bless both of you. She's in my constant thoughts and prayers.

Conversation with my sister-in-law.
⅃ Kim: Wow! I'm glad she's showing you this stuff. I'm sure it helps you to understand what's going on a little bit better. It sounds like she's in good hands!

⅃ Me: She's in the best hands for sure. She said Rachel must have been sick for a while.

⅃ Kim: Sounds like it. I'll check with you in the morning. Let me know if I can do anything.

7:16 pm, conversation with my sister.

↲ Colleen: Rachel is a fighter. I know she's
sedated but something in her is clearly fighting
and that can make a major difference. I feel like
a crappy sister for not getting up there today.

> ↲ Me: Rachel is fighting. That's the best sign of
> all. Don't feel that way. There's not much we can
> do right now but wait. You and George have
> always been there for us. My God, George went
> with me to Pennsylvania in the middle of the
> night when she had trouble. And you were with
> me through the whole mental hygiene attempt.
> Do you realize that was only like 4 months ago?!
> I really appreciate you both.

↲ Colleen: You know how much Rachel means to
us. We will always do anything we can for her.

> ↲ Me: I know that and I appreciate it more than I
> can say. The whole system is just so frustrating.
> I mean look at the mental hygiene thing. The
> police picked her up on a warrant filed by the
> landlord of that gross place she shared with RS.
> They called me at work to bail her out. The
> officer told me that she was really out of it and
> they found needles on her. On my way to the
> courthouse, it dawned on me that I could do
> something. I finally had an opportunity to take
> some action. It seemed meant to be, but it still
> took all of my nerve to try it.

↲ Colleen: Do you know if RS ever got arrested
on that warrant?

⌐ Me: Don't know. Don't care. I'm not sure if his name was on the lease. She got picked up because she had gone to school with the arresting officer. He saw her walking down the street and recognized her. He knew there was an outstanding warrant.

⌐ Colleen: I was kind of glad she got arrested. I was hoping for a turning point.

⌐ Me: Me too. I thought it might shake her up. I didn't realize how intense the proceedings were. I set it up with the officer and the magistrate. I bailed her out. While they processed that, I filled out the mental hygiene warrant. They released her to me then turned around and re-arrested her. I felt so mean. She was screaming. She looked at me and said "How could you do this to me?" I was shaking and trying not to cry.

⌐ Colleen: I'm really glad I wasn't there for that. I would have lost it.

⌐ Me: You wouldn't have liked the hearing part either. They first had us each talk to a psychologist separately. Then we waited for the judge to come and call us in. Rachel was at a table with the attorney they assigned to her. I was at a table on the other side by myself. I had to testify by myself and try to prove that she was a danger to herself. Then the psychologist gave his report. He backed up a lot of what I said. I think that was a big help. It was so nerve-wracking.

⌐ Colleen: I really don't know how you did it.

⌐ Me: I think I was just so desperate. The judge agreed with me that she needed help and ordered her to treatment. I was so relieved and so hopeful.

⌐ Colleen: I was too. So was George. That's why we went with you to visit her in that hospital. We were hoping that she might listen to us, figuring that she was mad at you.

⌐ Me: I know. You all were great. The problem is no one else cared, meaning that hospital. They knew exactly how long they were required to hold her in order to get paid, 72 hours which is a joke. They did nothing to help her. Withdrawing can be dangerous, I was shocked that they did not do anything for her. They just shuffled her out as fast as they could so they could get more money. Had she been treated better, she may have been more willing to continue with treatment at a better facility. I pinned so much hope on it. It was such a let-down.

⌐ Colleen: I know. It seemed like a lot of stress for nothing. I was so nervous when we went to pick her up. I thought she was going to be really mad, but she was so sweet. She hugged me.

⌐ Me: I remember. She knew that we acted out of love.

⌐ Colleen: I was hoping we would be able to reason with her and talk her in to going to that place that your doctor told you about.

⅃ <u>Me</u>: I know, me too. I'm just so aggravated thinking about things. There is so much talk about the opioid epidemic but when you actually try to take action there seems to be no urgency. We have a history of attempts. When she got back from the rehab in FL, she agreed to try a suboxone program. I knew we had to act quickly while she was detoxed and willing. I knew the longer we waited, the more likely she could relapse. I called immediately. I was told there was a waiting list for the program and they could not see her for 2 months. My heart sank.

⅃ <u>Colleen</u>: You have got to be kidding me!

⅃ <u>Me</u>: No, that is the reality of things. Rachel had another moment when I was able to reason with her. She agreed to an outpatient treatment. We walked in to the clinic and were treated with complete disregard. No one cared. We signed up on a sheet and waited and waited and waited. Rachel got more agitated with each passing hour. Finally after about 4 hours, we got called back to a room where we sat for a couple more hours getting absolutely nothing accomplished. No one was in a hurry. No one checked on us. We just sat. Finally, a "counselor" came in and said she could start treatment but she had to detox first. The problem was there were no beds available at any of the centers. So we sat. He looked at us, we looked at him and we just sat. I have no idea what the point was. Finally, Rachel just had enough, she was at her breaking point. She told him exactly what she thought and walked out. It was maddening.

⅃ <u>Colleen</u>: I don't blame her. That's heart breaking.

⤶ Me: I know, I don't get it. When an addict makes the giant step of being ready for treatment, they should be encouraged. There should be a process in place to take an immediate step. Start something, either talking or taking vital statistics. Keep them engaged and moving forward. Many of them already feel bad about themselves but then to get treated like they don't matter by supposed professionals is inexcusable.

⤶ Colleen: I'm glad I spent a couple hours online today researching heroin addiction and learning what kind of treatment facilities there are that would truly be able to help her. I want to be able to help her in any way I can.

⤶ Me: Thank you for checking that out because as she gets stronger we need to have something lined up.

⤶ Me: I'm also going to try to get her vivitrol. It's supposed to be like a miracle drug for opioid addicts. Look it up. It seems amazing.

DAY 10 Saturday, September 16, 2017

10:44 am, conversation with my sister-in-law.

⌐ Kim: How's it going today?

> ⌐ Me: About the same. She has a fever and her heart rate is up a little. I met the resident doctor this morning. He said they are just keeping her comfortable and giving her a lot of antibiotics until surgery. He thinks it will be this upcoming week.

⌐ Kim: That's good that there's a plan. How are you holding up?

> ⌐ Me: Pretty good. I think she's in the best hospital with the best doctors that will give her the best chance.

⌐ Kim: I agree! I don't know if I mentioned that we are in contract on our house. We are trying to get it empty. Still have a ton of stuff here to move. I'm not sure we'll get down there today, but please let me know if you need anything!

> ⌐ Me: I will. Thanks. That's exciting about your house but that's a lot of work!

⌐ Kim: Yes, and we're going out of town next Friday, which I hate with everything going on with Rachel.

> ⌐ Me: You know I will keep you posted. It seems like that's the way it works. Everything happens at once.

⌐ Kim: I know. Let us know if there's any change. Thx.

12:04 pm, conversation with a friend.
⌐ Me: I can't get the WVU game here.

⌐ Beth: I'll keep you posted. But this probably won't be a good one. Probably like last week. We are getting ready to score.......TD!!!

⌐ Me: Woo hoo!!! My dad just got here and found the game! I didn't scroll far enough on the channels!

⌐ Beth: Wow! It's not that hard to use a remote! Lol!

⌐ Me: Lol! Maybe not for you! I'm just glad he found it. I want Rachel to hear the game. She's not a huge football fan but she loves WVU since she went there. I was wearing a WVU jacket one of her first days in the hospital and she said she wanted it!

⌐ Beth: That will be nice for her to hear the game and have your dad there.

⌐ Me: I agree. Lightens the mood some!

12:29 pm, conversation with another friend.
⌐ Nancy: I just got home from fall decorating.....do you mind if we make lunch...dinner? How's Rachel? Any news on tests?

⌐ Me: She's about the same. I talked to one doctor but not the surgeon. I think they are planning on surgery next week.

⌐ Nancy: Good...I'll come around 5.

1:53 pm
⌐ Beth: So do you have any updates for me?

75

ↄ Me: No. She's been a little more awake today. She has opened her eyes and obeys commands. At this point stable is good!

ↄ Beth: YES!!! It certainly is!

ↄ Me: I should say she obeys commands when it suits her. She's still Rachel!

ↄ Beth: 😂😂😂! Omg! Funny. I about peed my pants! But so true!

ↄ Beth: I was thinking about what you told me the other day about going to PA to pick Rachel up. How did she ever get to NJ to begin with?

ↄ Me: After she and RS broke up, and she had been through the detox clinic, she moved in with a friend of hers. For whatever reasons, that didn't work out so she came home. She got a job at the Italian restaurant. She loved working there. She said she liked that she got to move around a lot and talk to people. She really liked the instant gratification of tips. She worked there for a while.

ↄ Beth: I know. I thought she was there but all of a sudden she was in NJ.

ↄ Me: She was picking up every open shift she could get. She didn't have a car so I would drop her off and usually one of her co-workers would bring her home. As she made friends there, she would spend the night with them. One of them lived close to the restaurant. She said it was easier. I didn't see her a lot. I thought working a lot and staying busy was helping her with everything she had been through. The red flag I see now is that she was always broke.

⌐ Beth: Do you think she was using again?

⌐ Me: I'm sure of it, but she always had an excuse. She would say she was paying back the people she stayed with. Plus she always did like to spend money. She is an adult so I couldn't really say much. I asked her, but she denied it. I went through her room but found no evidence.

⌐ Beth: There's not much else you can do, especially with no evidence.

⌐ Me: I guess that's kind of what I thought at the time. I also thought that she had already been through a lot. I didn't want her to think I didn't trust her. Things look much different now looking back than they did at the time.

⌐ Beth: For sure.

⌐ Me: She had been working at the restaurant for almost a year when she called me one night and said she had left West Virginia and was on her way to Ohio with her "team" for training. She said she was with a group that was going to travel across the country trying to get people to buy smart phones. It sounded very strange. I told her that too. I also told her I was worried for her safety. She assured me she was fine. She said she was excited to get to travel and see the country. She promised to keep in touch and let me know where she was and what she was doing. Every bad instinct alarm in me was going off, but she is an adult and she was already gone.

↲ Beth: Not selling smart phones? Trying to get people to buy smart phones? That definitely sounds strange. You couldn't really call the police or anything. She is an adult and she told you where she was, so it's not like she was abducted.

↲ Me: I know. I hated it. She ended up going with that group to NJ. She kept in touch but then a couple of weeks went by and she wasn't responding to my texts or calls. I was getting panicked. Finally she called me. There had been some sort of fight within the group and they booted her out. Literally, threw her out and left. It was the middle of the night and she was sick. She found a policeman and he took her to the hospital. She said she was dehydrated and had a fever. When she got released a girl she had met and the girl's boyfriend picked her up from the hospital and moved her in with them. I begged her to come home. She said she would eventually but she was going to stay there a while.

↲ Beth: From what you already told me, I know this was not good. Is this the situation she was trying to get away from when she called you hysterical that morning?

⅃ Me: Yes. You really don't want to know all of the details, but I do understand why she was desperate to leave. When we got back from PA, she was a mess not just from her addiction issues, but from a hygiene issue. She had not showered in 6 months. She always kept her hair in a sloppy bun on top of her head. It had been piled up there for so long untouched and unwashed that is was stuck. It was a giant matted mass on top of her head. I took her to a couple of salons to see if there was anything they could do but nobody would touch it. I ended up having to cut it out myself. I pulled out as much of her hair as I could then just cut the whole mass out. She had enough hair to frame her face and I cut the rest to shoulder length. When she wore a thick head band or pulled the sides up it really didn't look that bad.

⅃ Beth: I know. You sent me a picture of the hair mass! It was lovely!

⅃ Me: You're welcome for that btw! At that point she was running out of the withdrawal medicine they gave her in PA. She was very tired and weak. She agreed to a check-up with our family doctor. Her doctor was amazing. She told us that she has a brother that had addiction issues. She knew just how to talk to Rachel. She not only talked her in to going to rehab, she had a facility on the phone with plans already made before she even called me back. We left for Florida the next day.

2:21 pm

⤶ Me: The resident intern was looking at her. Everything's about the same. They gave her something to keep her comfortable and she is really out! The nurse said something that made me think. It's the least of the worries right now but he can't get her to use her left hand to squeeze, just the right. She has several small strokes. Maybe there's an issue from those.

⤶ Nancy: And that chunk of growth that traveled to her brain, too.

⤶ Me: Yes. I mean we will deal with whatever. That's a minor concern to me.

⤶ Nancy: True…

⤶ Me: As much as I would like to talk to her, I'm kind of glad they're keeping her comfortable. Every time she starts to wake up, she kind of fights the breathing tube. I'm guessing she doesn't like it.

⤶ Nancy: I imagine it's uncomfortable.

⤶ Me: Probably and kind of scary if you're groggy.

4:41 pm
⤶ Me: I did so good. I took a break and went to Gabes. I was looking for a WVU jacket for Rachel, but I found 4 pair of long women's pajama pants. Perfect for her as she recovers!

⤶ Beth: Good for you! You NEED breaks. Yes, she'll need them. What did you get for yourself?

⤵ Me: I wasn't shopping for me. That store is over whelming. It's easier if I stay on task! I was thrilled with those pants because they were only $5 each!

⤵ Beth: Whoa!!! Heck of a deal! Surprised you found them that cheap this time of year. I mean with cool weather coming.

⤵ Me: Finding talls was the bigger surprise!

⤵ Beth: Lol! True that!

⤵ Me: I wasn't sure what size to get. She's so skinny now, I got 2 pair of smalls. I got the other 2 medium because I remember when she came back from the rehab in FL she had gained some weight and a lot of her clothes were too tight.

⤵ Beth: I hope she does put on some weight. She needs it.

⤵ Me: I agree. I hope by the time she's ready for rehab this time, she will have already gained some.

⤵ Beth: I'm sure she will as she starts to feel better.

⤵ Me: Then I will happily go shopping again for new clothes. When she came back from NJ, she had nothing. It was October here and getting cool. I had to buy her a few things right away, warm clothes. Then she left for rehab in FL and it was so hot and humid there. I sent her several care packages with summer type clothes. She also asked for snack foods and candy!

⤵ Beth: My kind of girl!

ᒾ Me: Lol! I know. When she returned and I picked her up at the airport, I was surprised at how good she looked. She had been so gaunt before she left. It was so good to see her a little bit filled out. And her humor had returned. She was so funny. She did an impression of herself after medication disbursement time that had Maddy and I rolling!

ᒾ Beth: It seems like she did well there. Why did she leave?

ᒾ Me: I really don't know. She basically rejected what they were trying to teach her. It took a while for her to get adjusted. Once she did, she made some good friends. She had individual and group therapy. I did conference calls with her and her counselor for family therapy. Maddy and I sent impact letters when we were asked to. It started off good.

ᒾ Beth: We know it often takes more than 1 try at rehab.

ᒾ Me: I definitely know that. As she progressed, she was allowed more and more freedom. One day she just walked away. You know how strong willed she is. She does not like people telling her what to do. That may have something to do with it. I will never forget them calling me and telling me she left. I was freaking out because they didn't know where she was, but they were just notifying me that by leaving she was kicked out of the program.

ᒾ Beth: I remember. You were getting ready to fly out there.

↲ Me: I was going to find her and file a mental hygiene warrant there. They have much stricter laws in FL that would have kept her in treatment longer. When she finally contacted me, I knew she would take off if she suspected what I wanted to do. I thought it was more important to know where she was and have open communication with her, so I just flew her home. Knowing that she has to be ready to accept treatment, I didn't think it would do any good to force it on her. I still wonder if that was a mistake.

6:54 pm, conversation with my sister.
↲ Me: Not much to report today. She has had a persistent fever. They are giving her antibiotics and keeping her comfortable. Hopefully getting her ready for surgery soon.

↲ Kelly: I talked to Dad. He told me he visited today. He said things seem stable right now.

↲ Me: Yes. I'll take it! I did a little shopping, watched the WVU game and Nancy came today too.

↲ Kelly: That's nice. Sounds like you had a good day.

↲ Me: As a good a day as you can have in a hospital!

↲ Kelly: Lol! You know what I mean!

↲ Me: I know! Not as stressful today thankfully!

8:32 pm

↲ Me: I left the hospital a little early tonight. Not much has changed except that the nurse noticed today that Rachel would only respond on her right side. She didn't use her left side at all. That may be a result of the strokes. They will be checking her for that. All things considered that's a minor concern.

↲ Beth: Yes, it is. At this point, I'll take "not much has changed". Have they tried to remove her from the ventilator again?

↲ Me: No. They're not going to prior to surgery.

↲ Beth: Oh. Ok. Good

↲ Me: It's been a decent, uneventful day and that's a good thing. Whenever we have a quiet day and keep everything stable, it's a success!

↲ Beth: True!

8:48 pm, conversation with my sister-in-law.
↲ Kim: We are still at it over here. Lots more to do tomorrow. Would you like me to go down to the hospital in the morning for a little while before we get started?

↲ Me: Only if you want to. I don't want anyone to ever feel like they have to especially when you already have a ton on your plate. Right now all we can do is watch her breathe.

↲ Kim: Ok thanks. I'll let you know if I'm going.

DAY 11, Sunday, September 17, 2017

7:53 am, conversation with my sister-in-law.
Kim: Good Morning. I'm going to the hospital in about an hour, maybe sooner.

> Me: Ok. That's probably close to when I'm going. I took Zeppelin for a walk this morning so I'm a little behind.

Kim: If you need to do anything. I'll be happy to sit with her and send you an update!

> Me: I appreciate it. My main goal today was to walk Z so I'm good.

Kim: Ok. I'll see you soon then.

9:30 am
Kim: How soon will you be here? Doctors need to update you.

> Me: On my way

10:57 am, conversation with a friend.
Nancy: Are you at the hospital?

Nancy: Rick passed over this morning 🙏

> Me: Rachel took another turn for the worse.

Nancy: I'm coming!

12:12 pm, message to group.

↲ Me: I need to tell you what's happening. Rachel took a major turn for the worse. We are waiting for CT scan results. If it is ok she will be taken by helicopter to the University of Kentucky hospital for her only chance of survival. If it is bad, we just keep her comfortable until she dies. I don't know what else to say. That is the situation.

Conversation with a friend.

↲ Beth: Sorry. I lost you. For one of the few times in my life I'm at a loss for words. I didn't get all of it. I got the gist that she had a stroke and if CT scan shows it's bad, then they'll just keep her here and comfortable. But if not, they are flying her to UK. I feel so helpless. Whatever you want, I'll do. Love and prayers. They might not allow non family members there, but if so and you want me there, just say the word. In any case, please keep me updated.

↲ Me: Thanks. We are just waiting. I'll let you know. From what the surgeon said, they could do the surgery here, but they don't have the equipment or staff for the after surgery care she will need. He tried to explain things in terms I would understand. With each heartbeat, the infectious growth is spraying blood clots throughout her body. The CT scan will show if a large clot went to her brain. If so, she is no longer a candidate for the heart surgery. If she has the surgery, she will need a special machine, echmo or something like that, and they will have to leave her chest open for a while.

↲ Beth: Wow! I just put I had unspoken prayer request on my FB and my agnostic brother, having no clue as to what it was for, immediately liked it. I believe in the power of prayer. I know I said I feel helpless, but I do believe in prayers.

⅃ <u>Me</u>: I do too. Thanks!

12:15 pm
Response from my sister.
⅃ <u>Colleen</u>: I'm coming up there.

Conversation with my niece.
⅃ <u>Gaby</u>: If you're up for having visitors let me know and I'll come whenever.

⅃ <u>Gaby</u>: If there is anything I can do to help you let me know.

⅃ <u>Me</u>: I appreciate it. Aunt Kim, Nancy and my dad are here. We are just waiting.

⅃ <u>Gaby</u>: I'll be there in a few minutes.

⅃ <u>Me</u>: We are in the cafeteria right now. We will be going back up to the room in a few.

⅃ <u>Gaby</u>: Ok. Thank you. Can I bring anything?

⅃ <u>Me</u>: No but thanks.

1:13 pm, conversation with a work friend.
⅃ <u>Judy</u>: Oh, Maureen. Please keep me updated. I am praying.

⅃ <u>Me</u>: Thanks. I will. I'm praying too. That's all I know to do right now.

1:40 pm, conversation with my sister.
⅃ <u>Kelly</u>: I'm here whatever you want or need. I don't have words to be able to express what I want to say. If there's anything you need.

⅃ <u>Me</u>: Thanks. Still waiting. You could take Colleen off my hahds!

⅃ <u>Kelly</u>: Oh lord! What is she doing?

⌐ Me: You know what she does. She's getting all hysterical and it's really stressing me out worse! Dad just took her out of the room. Thank God!

⌐ Kelly: Oh good. Are you OK?

⌐ Me: I'm really nervous. I don't mean to get upset with Colleen, I'm just on edge.

⌐ Kelly: Of course you are. We all are.

⌐ Me: There's actually a support army in here! Dad, Kim, Nancy, Gaby, George and Colleen. I hope Rachel can feel all the love.

⌐ Kelly: I bet she can.

⌐ Me: Nancy brought a prayer blanket that some of the women at her church made. It's so nice. It has cats on it! The nurse laid it over Rachel's legs. It's comforting.

⌐ Kelly: That's so sweet. I'm glad it's helping.

⌐ Me: It is. I don't know if there is a limit to the number of people that are supposed to be here, but they haven't said anything! I'm sure they understand the need for support.

2:04 pm
⌐ Me: The resident doctor finally came in to talk to us. I don't think he realized we have been waiting all day on CT results. He said based on what he sees, there is no reason she can't make the trip! We are just waiting on a bed to open in any of the UK ICU's! I'm so happy but so nervous!

◁ Kelly: Oh thank God! I'm sure you're nervous but it's a good sign that she is going!

▷ Me: I know! That's what I think! It's the answer to all of the prayers today!

2:10 pm, conversation with a friend.
▷ Me: The doctor just said Rachel is good to go to UK!

◁ Beth: Hallelujah! When does she go? Do you know when the surgery will be?

▷ Me: We are just waiting on a bed to open up then she will be airlifted. I don't know about the surgery, but I'm sure ASAP.

3:36 pm, conversation with my daughter.
◁ Maddy: Are u riding with Rachel in the helicopter?

▷ Me: No. I don't think I'm allowed.

◁ Maddy: Okk

▷ Me: I'll be home before I leave.

◁ Maddy: Oh so ur leaving tonight?

▷ Me: If a bed opens up in any of the ICU's at UK. The surgeon said surgery should be done ASAP.

▷ Me: There is another issue today. She is not getting any blood flow to the lower part of her legs. Her feet are very cold and her toes are kind of purple. They have not been able to detect pulses in either leg.

◁ Maddy: What does that mean?

↲ Me: I'm not sure yet. They haven't really said.

4:05 pm, conversation with a work friend.
↲ Judy: Have they decided what they are planning to do?

↲ Me: A bed just opened up at the UK ICU. She will be air lifted out soon and my dad and I will follow by car. There is a chance the surgeon there will decide it's too risky to do surgery but this is her only chance.

↲ Judy: The ladies at Church will be praying for her and you about 5:30. Please be careful.

↲ Me: I will. Thanks. I'm shaking so hard I can barely type this.

↲ Judy: I can't even imagine. I am so glad your Dad is with you.

4:07 pm, message to group.
↲ Me: A bed just opened up at UK. She will be air lifted soon.

Conversation with a friend.
↲ Beth: As odd as it sounds, that is fantastic news!!!!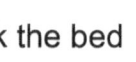

↲ Me: I know! I agree! I like to think the bed opened up for positive reasons!

↲ Beth: Me too!

Conversation with a friend.
↲ Nancy: Praise the Lord! Do you need me to drive you?

↲ Me: My dad is going to drive me. Thanks. Not sure what to do once I get there but we will figure it out!

⌐ Nancy: There is a sign for UK on I-64.

⌐ Me: Ok plus I have navigation.

⌐ Nancy: That'll be a plus!

Response from my sister-in-law.
⌐ Kim: Oh thank God! Please let me know if we can do anything. Keep me posted. Be safe!

Conversation with my niece.
⌐ Gaby: Excellent. The quicker the better.

⌐ Me: I agree!

4:54 pm
⌐ Me: So everyone has left. There were so many people here earlier. There was a lot of activity. It's really quiet now.

⌐ Kelly: When do you all leave?

⌐ Me: I'm waiting for the paramedics that will airlift her to get here. I don't want to leave her alone.

⌐ Kelly: I don't blame you. How are you? Do you have everything ready?

⌐ Me: Maddy is packing for me. I'm just going to run to an ATM, pick up my stuff, pick up dad and hit the road. I feel very anxious. Like things just keep happening and all I can do is watch. Out of control.

⌐ Kelly: I bet!

↲ Me: I'm looking at her now and it's like looking at baby Rachel. It's like she needs me and I just don't know what to do.

↲ Kelly: I understand that. She was our family's first baby. I think we all feel that way.

↲ Me: Definitely. This whole thing seems unreal. We all need to stick together and get her healthy in every way.

↲ Kelly: She has a lot of family that will be there for her.

↲ Me: Very true. A very large extended family. There are so many people that have reached out. And so many people like Beth, Nancy and Judy going through it with us.

↲ Kelly: Yes. I didn't just mean blood relatives! You know that you all are in my constant thoughts and prayers. Be careful. I love you both.

↲ Me: Thanks! Love you too! I'll keep you posted.

6:52 pm
↲ Nancy: Have you made it yet?

↲ Me: We're on our way.

7:43 pm
↲ Kim: Did she get out ok?

↲ Me: Yes. We are on our way now. They were supposed to call when she got there and I haven't heard anything yet.

↲ Kim: Ok great. Thanks 🙏

8:58 pm, conversation with my daughter.

⊣ Maddy: Did you make it ok?

⊣ Me: We are still on our way.

⊣ Me: PawPaw is not going to stay. He's going to help me get settled then is going to head back. You should come after the surgery while she's in recovery.

⊣ Maddy: Okk

9:23 pm

⊣ Nancy: 🙏 There is never "too late" 🩶

⊣ Me: I know! This is our Hail Mary pass! We've been given this for a reason!

10:26 pm

⊣ Me: We're here and we found Rachel! She's about the same and that's good that she's not worse.

⊣ Maddy: Okk Thank God! What's the situation with the surgery?

⊣ Me: We don't know yet.

⊣ Maddy: Okk keep me posted! How long is pawpaw staying?

⊣ Me: He's resting a few hours and going back. If we can make arrangements for Z, I would like you to be here. If you want to be.

⊣ Maddy: Yeaa I want to be there can I come up in the morning?

↲ Me: Absolutely. Beth said she could help with Z any time or MeeMaw.

↲ Maddy: Ok. I'll figure something out.

DAY 12, Monday, September 18, 2017

5:46 am, message to work friend.
↲ Me: Rachel passed away at about 3 a.m. this
morning. There really wasn't much they could do
here. The heart growth was spraying blood clots,
and she ended up having a brain hemorrhage.

EPILOGUE

My dad and I had been up for so long. As soon as the paramedics arrived to airlift Rachel, I left to quickly get organized and pack. I picked my dad up and we took my car. The trip seemed long. Upon arriving in Lexington, it took a while to find the University of Kentucky Hospital. It is a huge complex. All I had was a hand written note from the nurse at Memorial that said, "Pavilion A (new part), 10th Floor – tower 2, bed 233". It seems like we circled around for hours, but it was actually only about 20 minutes. We raced through the parking building and into the hospital. We found Rachel and she looked just like she had in West Virginia. That brought a huge feeling of relief. I was so happy to see her there.

The hospital was very nice. Her room was big and even had a place for us to rest. The view was incredible over-looking some of the UK campus. Everything was lit up. It was quite pretty and seemed very peaceful. The staff was polite and helpful.

Memorial Hospital had sent all of her records and test results on a CD. While the staff in KY was waiting for all of the tests to upload, they started examining her. Each doctor asked us a lot of questions. I was so tired it was hard to focus enough to answer. One of the first concerns was her legs. There was no blood flow to the lower parts of either leg. A doctor and some of her team examined them. They said they were going to do a few more tests and then try to address the problem. Different doctors and staff listened to her heart multiple times. The other big issue was her cognitive state. She was unresponsive. The staff already knew about some of the strokes and that her left side didn't respond to any stimulus. They mentioned doing a spinal tap at one point.

As soon as they were able to read the last CT scan that had been done, they sent a neurologist to talk to us. The scan showed evidence of brain trauma. She said that before anything else could be done, they needed to do an MRI to see how significantly the brain had been affected. I was able to stay at Rachel's bed side and talk to her until they came to take her for testing. They can do a lot of tests in the room, but not that one. It took a few people to move all of the equipment with her. My dad and I stayed in the room and tried to rest, but mostly talked.

About 30 minutes later, they brought her back. It felt to me like there was a whirlwind of activity. There were doctors and nurses coming in and out. They were talking. There were machines humming and beeping. The neurologist came to talk to us. She told us the facts. There was a lot of swelling in Rachel's brain. She had multiple lesions. The back part of the brain was starting to shift downward into the top of the spinal cord. This is called a brain herniation. There are things they could do to alleviate the pressure. She said that they could shave half of Rachel's head, drill a hole in her skull and drain some of the fluid. This would only prolong the process of complete herniation that was imminent. She continued that even with the procedure, the Rachel that we knew was already gone. At best, we would be preserving a body that would always need care and life support. My dad and I talked. We actually considered the procedure for a short while. Finally, my dad said, "this child has been through enough. It's time to let her be at peace". I agreed. A moment later, the nurse told us that Rachel had soiled the bed. He asked us to step out while he cleaned her up.

My dad and I were in kind of a stunned, bewildered state. We decided to go to the cafeteria. This would allow us to get away for a few minutes and try to process things. I was shaking and quietly crying. We found a booth and sat. I had a feeling of disbelief. I struggled with knowing during this time that Rachel was going to die. I didn't yet know the final details, but I knew there were no more options. It was achingly surreal.

I sat in uncertainty, desperate for something solid to grab a hold of. Just a few hours ago, Rachel's hospital room was full of people who dearly loved her. The energy in the room pulsated with love and hope. The reflection was broken when my phone suddenly rang. It was the nurse telling me that Rachel was already showing signs of herniation and we should return.

When we got back to the room, it was quiet. I could already see the difference. Rachel looked so small. Her breathing was hard. I could tell the ventilator was doing all of the work. I could see the motion of air being pushed into her lungs. The force of it rocked her body. The nurse explained to us that they were going to slowly start removing the life support equipment. A chaplain came in to talk to us. We said a prayer. The nurse asked if I wanted the heart monitor to be turned off. I don't know why, but I didn't. I liked being able to see the line arc with her heartbeat. He turned the volume off but left the screen on.

Finally, all of the machines were gone. I could see Rachel's face fully. I took her hand between mine. My dad put his hands over mine. We stood there watching as Rachel's breathing became shallow and less frequent. I was able to tell her that I loved her. The line on the heart monitor became flat. The nurse stepped back in to the room to tell us she was gone, but I already knew. Her pained expression had become serene. Rachel passed in just a few brief moments after the ventilator was removed.

I didn't want to let her hand go. Tears streamed uncontrollably down my face. My dad wept openly. The chaplain came back in for another prayer. The nurse returned with a beautiful picture of a tree with heart-shaped roots. He put each of Rachel's finger prints on it and handed it to me. He told us to take as long as we needed and left the room.

We sat in silent grief for a while. Finally, my dad suggested that we make some calls. We called family first, then a couple of close friends. I attempted to talk to a local funeral home but could not get any words out. My dad was able to take over and make the arrangements to bring Rachel back to West Virginia. After a flurry of blurred chaos with emotional extremes of high and low, the day was over. We headed home.

For Rachel

I don't know how to start this, my final message to you.
There's so much I want to say, so many questions too.
All I have are simple words, no eloquent way to express;
thoughts and feelings trapped in my mind on which I do
obsess.
From the start, you brought a feeling that could never sway;
no matter what, I love you. I'll be with you all the way.

Times are seldom simple, we had our share of strife. We
always kept on trying, knowing that's just part of life.
But drugs came in and took control, we were up against a
beast. From its cruel crippling grip, I could not will your
release.
You made such scary choices, to this day I don't know why.
Were you searching for your place? Did you care that you
might die?

So funny and endearing, now fallen far off track. I feel you
fighting for yourself. How do I get you back?
I went against my instincts with many different tries; intent to
make an impact, so you would realize.
Despite the pain and conflict, disease steadily advanced;
leaving only desperate longing for another chance.

Then came the day I got a call, your affliction came to light. I
had never heard of it. There is no way this could be right.
The facts about your illness did reveal a challenged plight.
Troubling, but I know my girl. She will fight with all her might.
I called in reinforcements, a family came together; united and
defiant against the murky weather.

Days went by and haze raged on, it made me feel quite
helpless. I could only watch and wait and wish to not be
useless.
As I sat, it made me ponder of what you were aware. Did you
dream? Could you hear? Did you know that I was there?
If only I could talk to you and hold you close and tight. I

wanted to protect you and make everything all right.

I tried to do the right things. What more could I have done?
Somehow I still failed you. From this I cannot run.
Do you forgive me? A painful question, an answer I won't get.
The bigger thing I want to know has the most significance yet.
When you acknowledged your mistakes, were you asking for
forgiveness? I would absolve you anything, but were you
seeking Godly witness?

Progression came so quickly, now an all-consuming hole.
Things just kept unraveling taking a perilous toll.
Struggling with the outcome of every crucial choice; through
the frenzied chatter, I strained to hear a guiding voice.
I prayed intensely day by day, but you kept fading further
away. I asked for healing free from pain; relief from the
relentless strain.

As a human being there is so little I control. I can only love
and hope from deep within my soul.
In the end, the Lord decides if we will live or die. Even though I
know it's wrong, I've started asking why.
The time had come. There is no way to ever be prepared. I
wish you strength, my daughter, I pray you were not scared.

There was nothing left to do but take your hand in mine;
trembling as I searched your face for any given sign.
The moment felt surreal. The tears they would not cease.
Forever in my mind I'll see your expression fade to peace.
It's not how I envisioned what my faith does clearly see, the
answer to so many prayers allowed you to be free.

I was there at the beginning, from your very first heartbeat. My
head now spinning from the speed of life to be complete.
I am striving to stay faithful and trying to embrace, allowing me
to be there was truly given grace.
I must still be in shock. I just can't comprehend, the futility of
things endured for such a brutal end.

Disheartened in the ending days by time to contemplate, what

your journey might have been had heroine not chosen your
fate.
Final is a massive block my mind can't get around. If we could
do things over, would the answers be found?
Life is always teaching; of all the things I've learned, the
harshest of these lessons are the ones that remain yearned.

There is a tender twilight that keeps sanity protected. It
happens after all is lost, peace in feeling still connected.
Through those that knew your true self, your spirit remains
here. With every breath I ever take, you will still be near.
I hope you know the things that will stay eternally true. You will
always have my love. I would have never given up on you.

www.ingramcontent.com/pod-product-compliance
Lightning Source LLC
Chambersburg PA
CBHW030949240526
45463CB00016B/2243